T
HE
ATOZ
OF EYES
INTRODUCTION

T0319304

...ack **appreciated**
medicalamanda@gmail.com

Acknowledgement

Thank you Aspen Pharmacare Australia for your support and assistance in this valuable project, particularly Greg Lan, Rob Koster, Richard Clement and Robbie Drew.

Dedication

To Greg Lan - this book is his suggestion.

How to use this book

The format of this A to Z book has been maintained. The Common terms section has been expanded and illustrated. Simple definitions and explanations along with many of the pathological opthalmic conditions are listed here. The first section - **The Eye – Adnexae, Components & Relations** lists the major components of the eye and its surroundings, in the A to Z way i.e. alphabetically. Of course in a unit such as this the structure may be demonstrated in a number of ways and with other structures, which is indicated where appropriate. The second section **The Eyes - Examination, Malfunction & Testing** focuses on common eye conditions, their presentations and causes. So as usual *think of it and then find it* is the motto of *the A to Zs*. Eyes are complex, and they cannot be considered without some optic theory which is included in the second section.

Please note also that additional material may be found in the other A to Zs: *the A to Z of the Brain and Cranial Nerves, the A to Z of Major Organs* and *the A to Z of Hair, Nails & Skin* in particular.

For an interactive educational Ophthalmic App, visit the App store and search Aspen Eye. Password: ophthalmics

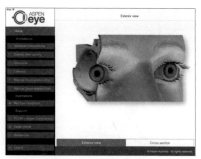

Thank you
A. L. Neill
BSc MSc MBBS PhD FACBS

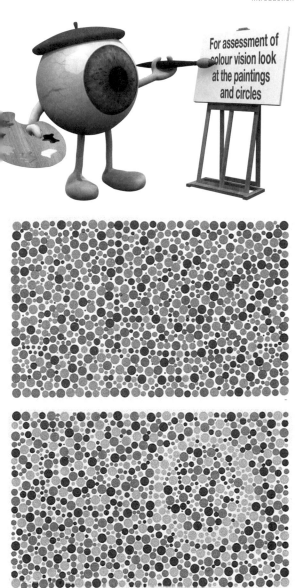

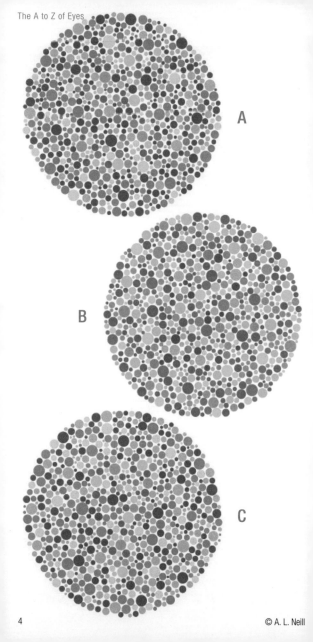

A

B

C

4

D

E

F

Answers

a brown boat
a yellow circle + a brown square
A: 5, B: 2, C: 7, D: 6, E: 10, F: 57

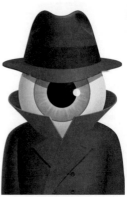

To further check on eye function - stare at the centre of this Amsler grid, with one eye, wearing glasses or CLs if needed. If all the lines are not visible, even & straight, and the grid is not rectangular & clear see the *Visual Acuity Assessment*.

Similarly the Astigmatic clock should also appear to have even, regular straight spokes. MT p286 for assessment.

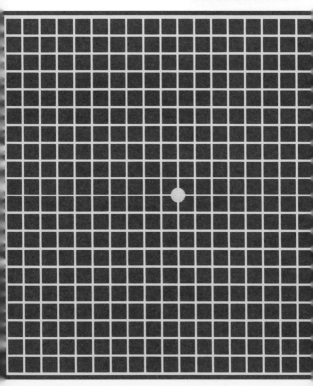

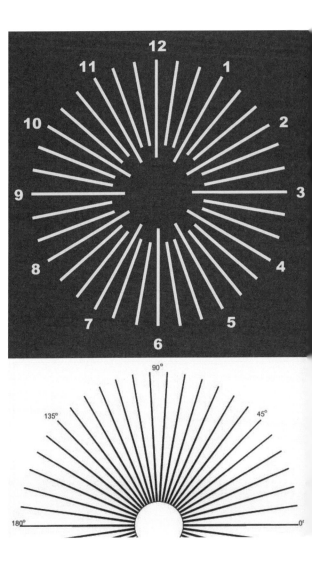

TABLE OF CONTENTS

The Eye – Adnexae, Components & Relations

The Eyes - Examination, Malfunction & Testing

Abbreviations, Acronyms & Symbols

Note these abbreviations include those in common use in the study and examination of the eyes as well as the ones used in this book

A

a	= artery
aa	= anastomosis (ses)
AA	= amino acid
Ab	= antibody
AC	= anterior chamber
ACG	= acute angle glaucoma
ACTH	= adrenocorticotropic hormone / adrenal cortical hormone
ADH	= antidiuretic hormone
adj.	= adjective
ADP	= adenosine diphosphate
ADV	= adenovirus
Ag	= antigen
AH	= aqueous humour
AI	= autoimmune
AKA	= also known as
alt.	= alternative
AMD	= age-related macular degeneration
AMP	= adenosine monophosphate
ANS	= autonomic nervous system
ant.	= anterior
AO	= adult onset
AODM	= adult onset diabetes mellitus
AS	= Alternative Spelling, generally referring to the diff. b/n British & American spelling
ATP	= adenosine triphosphate
av	= arterial-venous / arteriole-venule

B

B	= blood
b	= bone
bb	= basal bodies
BBB	= blood-brain-barrier
bc	= because
BCC	= basal cell carcinoma
BDR	= background diabetic retinopathy
BM	= basement membrane / basal lamina / terminal lamina / plasma lamina
b/n	= between
BP	= blood pressure
br	= branch
BS	= Blood Supply / blind spot
BStem	= brain stem

C

CB	= ciliary body
Ch	= choroid
Ci	= cilium (a)
CC	= cerebral cortex
C/D	= cup to disc ratio
c.f.	= compared to
CG	= ciliary ganglion
CH	= cerebral hemispheres
CL	= contact lens
CM	= cellular membrane / plasma membrane
CN	= cranial nerve
CNS	= central nervous system
CNV	= choroidal neovascularization
Co	= collagen

CP	= cervical plexus		**Es**	= eyelash
collat.	= collateral		**E-W**	= Edinger-Westphal nucleus
Cr	= cranial			
CSF	= cerebrospinal fluid		**ext.**	= extensor (as in muscle to extend across a joint)
CT	= connective tissue / computed tomography			
CTR	= common tendinous ring			

F

D			**F**	= fibre
			FB	= foreign body
D	= diopter / detachment		**FEM**	= fast eye movements
DD	= differential diagnosis		**Fi**	= filament / fibril
DES	= dry eye syndrome		**FHx**	= family history
DF	= Decemet's fold		**FP**	= foot process / focal point
diff.	= difference(s)		**FS**	= fibrous sheath
dist.	= distal		**FUO**	= fever of unknown origin
DM	= diabetes mellitus / dura mater		**FVP**	= fibrovascular proliferation
DNA	= deoxyribonucleic acid			
DOPA	= dihydroxyphenylalanine		**G**	
DT	= digestive tract		**GA**	= Golgi apparatus
DVM	= optic disc + retinal blood vessels + macula		**GCL**	= ganglion cell layer (of the retina)
Dx	= diagnosis		**gen.**	= generally
			GH	= growth hormone
E			**gld**	= gland
			Gk.	= Greek
E	= energy / eye		**GM**	= grey matter
EAM	= external acoustic meatus		**Gr**	= granule
EB	= eyeball			
ec	= extracellular		**H**	
e.g.	= example			
EL	= eyelid		**h**	= hour
ELM	= external limiting membrane (of the retina)		**H**	= hormone
			HA	= headache
EM	= eye movements		**Hb**	= haemoglobin
EMD	= exudative macular degeneration		**HBP**	= high blood pressure
			HCL	= hard contact lens
EO	= extraocular		**H&E**	= haematoxylin & eosin
EOM	= extraocular muscles		**Hg**	= haemorrhage
epi.	= epithelium		**HP**	= high pressure
ER	= endoplasmic reticulum		**HR**	= heart rate

HS	= Herpes Simplex
HTN	= hypertension
Hx	= history

I

IAM	= Internal acoustic meatus
ic	= intracellular (inside the cell)
ICP	= intracranial pressure
If	= inflammation
Ig	= immunoglobulin
IHD	= ischaemic heart disease
IIL	= idiopathic intracranial hypertension
In	= infection
INL	= inner nuclear layer (of the retina)
int.	= internal
IO	= intraocular / Inferior Oblique muscle
IOM	= intraocular muscles
IOP	= intra-ocular pressure
IPD	= interpupillary distance
IPL	= inner plexiform layer (of the retina)
IR	= inflammatory reaction/ response / Inferior Rectus muscle
IT	= inferior turbinate (of the nose)
IV	= intravenous

J

Jc	= junctional complex
jt(s)	= joints = articulations

K

KP	= keratic precipitate

L

l	= lymphatic
L	= lumbar / left
LA	= lacrimal apparatus
LE	= left eye
llg	= ligament
LL	= lower limb / lower eyelid
LP	= lamina propria
LPS	= Levator Palpebrae Superioris muscle
LR	= Lateral Rectus muscle
LT	= lymphoid tissue
Lt.	= Latin
LIF	= left iliac fossa
LUQ	= left upper quadrant

M

m	= muscle
M	= macula / magnification
MA	= microaneurysm
MD	= macular degeneration
med.	= medial
mem	= membrane
MH	= macular hole
MI	= myocardial infarction / heart attack
M-G	= Marcus- Gunn pupil
mito	= mitochondrion (a)
MM	= mucus membrane / millimeters
mmHG	= millimeters of mercury (pressure)
MNC	= mononuclear cells
monos	= monocytes
MR	= Medial Rectus muscle
MRA	= magnetic resonance angiography
MRI	= magnetic resonance imaging
mRNA	= messenger RNA

mt	= microtubule		**ONH**	= optic nerve head
MT	= main text		**ONL**	= outer nuclear layer (of the retina)
mu	= muscle		**OO**	= orbicularis oculi
mv	= microvillus (i)		**OP**	= ocular pressure (of the EB)
MVR	= massive vitreous retraction		**ophthal.**	= ophthalmology / ophthalmic
			OPL	= outer plexiform layer (of the retina)

N

n	= noun		**OS**	= left eye (oculus sinister)
N (s)	= nerve(s)		**OU**	= both eyes
N/A	= not applicable		**OZ**	= optical zone
Na	= sodium			
NAD	= normal (size, shape)			

P

NAD	= no abnormality detected		**PaNS**	= parasympathetic nervous system
NFL	= nuclear fibre layer (of the retina)		**PC**	= posterior chamber / posterior commissure
NLD	= nasolacrimal duct		**PERL**	= pupils equal and reactive to light
NM	= nuclear membrane / nucleolemma		**pH**	= measure of alkalinity / acidity of a solution
No	= nucleolus		**PH**	= pinhole visual acuity / past history
Np	= nuclear pore		**pl.**	= plural
NP	= near point		**PN**	= peripheral nerve
NR	= nerve root origin		**PNS**	= peripheral nervous system
NS	= nerve supply / nervous system / normal saline		**prn**	= as required / as needed (pro re nita)
NT	= nervous tissue		**post.**	= posterior
Nu	= nucleus		**proc.**	= process
nv	= neurovascular bundle		**prox.**	= proximal
NV	= neovascularization / near vision			

R

NVM	= neovascular membrane		**R**	= right / resistance

O

O	= origin (gen. muscle)		**RBC**	= red blood cell
OA	= over active (gen. muscle)		**RD**	= retinal detachment
OD	= optic disc		**Re**	= retina
OD	= right eye (oculus dexter) - not used here as a ref only		**RE**	= refractive error
ON	= optic nerve			

13

RF	= refractive index		**supf**	= superficial
RNA	= ribonucleic acid		**sv**	= synaptic vesicle
			SymNS	= sympathetic nervous system
rRNA	= ribosomal RNA			
RP	= refractive power			
RPE	= retinal pigmented epithelium			

T

T	= tissue
tab	= tablet
TED	= thyroid eye disease
TIA	= transient ischaemic attacks
Tm	= tumour
TNF	= tumour necrosis factor
TNTC	= too numerous to count
TP	= tarsal plates
tRNA	= transfer RNA / transport RNA
tu	= tubule
tw	= terminal web
Tx	= treatment / therapy

RUQ = right upper quadrant

S

s	= without (sine)
sc	= subcutaneous / w/o visual aids
SC	= spinal cord
SCC	= squamous cell carcinoma
SCL	= soft contact lens
SD	= standard deviation
SEM	= slow eye movements
sep	= separation
SI	= small intestine
sig	= instructions (signeteur)
sing.	= singular
SL	= Schwalbe's line
SMD	= senile macular degeneration
SN	= spinal nerve
SO	= Superior Oblique muscle
SOB	= shortness of breath
SOF	= superior orbital fissure
soln	= solution
SOV	= superior orbital vein
SR	= Superior Rectus muscle
SRH	= subretinal haemorrhage
SRM	= subretinal membrane
ss	= signs & symptoms / scleral spur
subcut.	= subcutaneous (just under the skin)

U

UA	= underactive (muscle)
UCVA	= uncorrected visual acuity
UL	= upper limb / upper eyelid
ULC	= upper eyelid crease
ung	= ointment (unguentum)

V

V	= vein
v	= very
va	= vacuole
vb	= verb
VA	= visual acuity
VAA	= visual association areas
VB	= vitreous body
VECP	= visually evoked cortical potential

VEGF	= vascular endothelial growth factor
VER	= visual evoked response
VF	= visual field
VH	= vitreous haemorrhage
Vi	= virus
VL	= vision loss / loss of vision
VP	= visual pathway
vs	= vesicle
VMT	= vitreomacular traction
VOD	= vision of the right eye
VOR	= vestib-ocular reflex
VOS	= vision of the left eye
VOU	= vision of both eyes
VZV	= varicella zoster virus

W

WM	= white matter
w/n	= within
w/o	= without
wrt	= with respect to

X

X	= exophoria / power of magnification

YZ

ZA	= zonula adherans
ZO	= zonula occludens / tight junction

Symbols

&	= and
#	= fracture
↓	= decreased / depressed
↑	= increased / elevated
>	= greater than
<	= less than
∩	= intersection with
≠	= opposite of / unequal to

Pronunciation Key & Colour Guide

Most terms are listed in black.

Pathological terms are in green

Prefixes and Suffixes are in blue

The pronunciation guide to words in this section are in bold red lettering

Stressed syllables are in **CAPITAL LETTERS**

Vowel sounds are pronounced as indicated below

A	May	ay
	map	a
	mark	ah
E	Me	ee
	met	e
	term	ur
I	eye / sight	ï
	tin	i
O	go	oh
	mother	uh
	mop	o
	more	or
	boy	oi
	lose	oo
	nook	oe
	loose	ou
U	blue	ou
	cute	ew
	cut	uh
Y	family	ee
	myth	i
	eye	ï

Common Terms used to describe the eyes; their structure & functions

A

ab externo surgical term to describe excisions which go from the outside to the inside

ab interno surgical term to describe excisions which go from the inside to the outside

Abduction movement away from the midline e.g. outward rotation of the eye from straight ahead (≠ **Adduction**)

Abducens AKA Abducent AKA Abducen N CN VI has the longest intracranial route of all the CNs

Aberration (ab-er-RAY-shon) blurred or distorted image quality results from internal physical properties of an optical device e.g. comma aberration when dots outside the optical axis appear as commas - a form of astigmatism *adj aberrant*

Aberrant unusual, abnormal

Aberrant regeneration functional defect e.g. the abnormal regrowth of a N after ly e.g. CN III br to the IR grows to the upper EL & causes it to rise when looking down instead of following the direction of the EB

Ablate remove or destroy surgically or radiologically *(n ablation)*

Ablepharon (a-BLEF-ar-on) absence of ELs

Abrasion removal of top layers of a structure in ly *see Corneal abrasion (vb abrade* - to scrape away a surface/ layer)

Acanthamoeba (ay-kan-thuh-MEE-buh) single cell MO protozoan found in the soil & contaminated water which causes keratitis with CLs

Accommodation ability to change the shape of the lens via the muscles of the CB to focus on close objects

Achromat AKA Monochromat an individual w/o the ability to distinguish b/n colours or who can only see 1 colour due to an absence of cones or only having one cone type

Achromatic lens lens to reduce chromatic aberration -splitting of colours

Actinic related to sun exposure

Acuity *see Visual acuity*

Adduction movement towards the midline e.g. inward rotation of the eye from straight ahead (≠ **Abduction**)

adeno- related to glands

Adonoid glandular

Adenopathy generally refers to the swelling of LNs due to In or IR

Adenovirus group of viruses causing: conjunctivitis, If of the mms, URTIs,

Adherence syndromes AKA Cicatricial strabismus AKA Johnson's syndrome syndromes which limit the movements of the eyes because of adhesions b/n the sheaths of EOM, post ly or trauma to the muscle cone

Adherent leukoma (LOO-koh-muh) dense corneal opacity to which the iris is attached, may or may not encroach upon the pupil

Adie's pupil AKA Pupillotonia AKA Tonic pupil ↓ pupillary constriction to light & sluggish redilatation, & poor accommodation for near objects – due to ly to the ciliary ganglion

Adjunctive Tx a Tx which enhances / assists the therapeutic effect of a medication or other Tx

Adjustable sutures used in the Tx of strabismus to adjust the attachment site of the EOMs in the fine tuning of the operation

Adjuvant Tx a Tx that enhances the body's response to a medication

Adnexa (ae) (AD-nex-a/ee) appendages & associated structures of the primary structure or organ *wrt eye* the EL, eyebrow, orbit & its contents *cf adnexae oculi*

Advancement the surgical reattachment of an EOM to a more forward position on the EB – to strengthen its action

Aerial haze atmospheric effects which give distant objects a blue haze - assists in monocular depth perception

Afebrile w/o fever *(≠ Febrile)*

Afferent pupillary defect AKA Gunn pupil AKA Marcus-Gunn pupil slow light reaction 2° to ON disease where there is slow conduction of the ON - Ex with the swinging flashlight

After-cataract an opacity developing after the removal of the lens - generally on the lens capsule *see also Elschnig pearls*

After-image an image which persists after 1 or both eyes are exposed to a bright light this phenomenon can be used to test if retinal correspondence is normal – using different images for each eye & determining the after-images of each

Age-related macular degeneration (AMD) a disease entity causing VL due to the dissociation &/or interruption of the retina from its BS in the macular region which ↑ with age *(see also Drusen, Macular Degeneration)*

Agnosia (ag-NOHZ-ee-uh) inability to recognize objects despite having an intact VP *see also Alexia*

Agonist / Primary mover *wrt eye* the main EOM responsible for the eye movement direction

Air/Fluid exchange *wrt eye* replacing the vitreous fluid with air or gas after Tx for retinal detachment *(see also vitrectomy)*

Alacrima lack of tear production

Albinism an hereditary condition with the absence of melanin pigment, which includes lack of pigment in the retina & iris comprising VA, bc of too much light w/n the EB.

Alexia word blindness with perfect vision (due to brain damage) *see also Agnosia*

Allen cards - picture cards used for the illiterate or children to examine VA *see also Snellen charts*

Alveolus (al-VEE-oh-lus) air filled cavity e.g. sinus *adj - alveolar* (as in air filled bone in the Frontal bone or Maxilla)

Amacrine cells AS Amarcrine long retinal neural cells of the IPL facilitating communication across & w/n the retina connecting the bipolar & ganglion cells

Amaurosis (am-uh-ROH-sus) AKA Leber's congenital amaurosis blindness or near-blindness due to ↓ retinal function possibly involving the amacrine or interconnecting cells of the INL.

Amaurotic pupil the pupil of a blind eye due to ON disease; it contracts in response to light only when the normal eye is stimulated with light, but the normal eye does not react when the amaurotic pupil is so stimulated.

Amblyopia *(adj amblyopic)* AKA Lazy Eye ↓ VA which cannot be explained by analysis of the VP; generally the vision of one eye is suppressed in favour of another due to the mal-alignment of the EOM

Types: **Ametropic/ Refractive** - large uncorrected RE in one or both eyes
    Anisometropic - large RE difference b/n the 2 eyes
    Deprivation / Occlusion/Disuse - loss of VA in an eye bc of loss of central fixation disuse, maybc 2° to Tx to enhance the VA in a deviated eye & so suppressing input from the normal eye, or some other obstruction to the retina e.g. cataract – reversed with removal of the deprivation form the incident light
    Hysterical - non-physiological cause usually presents as tunnel vision
    Meridonal - VA loss or reduction due to uncorrected astigmatism
    Nutritional /Toxic - due to Vita. B deficiency ± alcohol & drug
    Receptor - pathology in the rods &/or cones
    Strabismic - assoc with crossed eyes - cf inward deviation of one eye in childhood will suppress the input in that eye in favour of the eye which fixates centrally. This is reversible up to 9yo prior to maturation of the VP

Amsler grid graph image - with central dot, to use for assessment of MD (& AMD); if the waves either side of the dot appear wavy the eye may have MD *see also MT p286*

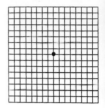

Anaemia AS anemia (an-EE-mee-ya) lack of haemoglobin detected by looking at the conjunctiva of the lower EL which is pale

Anatomic Equator *see Equator*

angio (anj-EE-oh) to do with BVs

Angiogenesis formation of new BVs

Angioscotoma blind spot due to the shadow of a retinal BV *see also Scotoma*

Angiography test used to examine the BVs using a dye; *wrt eyes* the ocular BS may be isolated & examined

Angle *of the eye* is the meeting place of the cornea & iris inside the eye, in the normal eye it must be open - closure results in an accumulation of AH & hence ↑ IOP

Anhidrosis absence of sweating

Anions negatively charged atoms or radicals e.g. Cl-, OH-

Aniridia congenital absence of the iris

Aniseikonia (an-is-EE-koh-ee-uh) different images perceived by each eye either in size shape or colour; may lead to Amblyopia

Anisocoria differences in the size of the 2 pupils

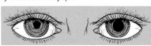

Anisometropia differences in the refractive errors b/n each eye

Annulus a peripheral ring surrounding an inner structure

Annulus of Zinn AKA Common Tendinous Ring (CTR) fibrous band that serves as an insertion point for the EOM resting on top of the orbital fissure; ON passes through the centre

Anophthalmos (an-OPFF-thal-mos) absence of a true EB

Anopsia VL of part of the VF

Anton's syndrome condition where patient still believes they can see despite the destruction of the visual cortex

Antioxidants substances external or synthesized in the body, which protect cells from oxidative damage due to free radicals

Aperture an opening or space b/n bones or w/n a bone.

Aphakia (AY-FAYK-ee-uh) absence of a crystalline lens

　　　© A. L. Neill

Apocrine secretions in which the cytoplasm of the apex of the cell is shed as well

Aqueous clear watery fluid c.f. the fluid which fills the ant. & post. chambers in the eye

Aqueous flair AKA Tyndall effect scattering of the slit lamp rays in the ant. chamber due to ↑ protein assoc. with lf of the ant. chamber contents e.g. iritis

Arachnodactyly (uh-rak-noh-DAK-til-ee) AKA Marfan's syndrome CT disease characterized by long thin appendages, relaxed ligs, loose jts & congenital heart disease, *wrt eyes*: cataracts, incomplete choroid formation, large corneas, dislocated lenses, ↑ myopia, ptosis & strabismus

Arc curve *adj arcuate*

Arc of contact AKA Contact Arc distance b/n the contact & insertion of the EOMs on the sclera of the EB see also Spiral of Tillaux

Arcades arches *wrt eye*: normal pattern of retinal BVs which arch in a circle around the macula & iris

Arcus Senilis AKA Gerontoxon a grey / cream ring around the limbus in the cortex occuring in those >60yo, or in those with elevated fat levels

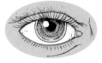

Arcus Juvenilis a similar condition in the young

Arden plates AKA Contrast sensitivity test grey cards with image & backgrounds with minimal difference in shading to detect the ability to discriminate subtle gradations b/n image & target – primarily the function of the rod cells in peripheral vision *see also MT p284*

Area Centralis clinical term for the Macula Lutea *see Macula*

Areola small, open spaces c.f. the areolar part of the Maxilla may lead or develop into sinuses.

Argyll-Robertson pupil AKA light–near disassociation small unequal pupils that constrict for near focus but do not react to light assoc. with BStem lesions *see also Dorsal midbrain syndrome*

Asteroid Hyalosis degen. process - small Ca deposits in the VB - no VL *see also Synchysis Scintillans*

Asthenopia eye fatigue / eye discomfort

Astigmatism a RE characterized by the irregular curvature of the cornea &/or lens which distorts the image & does not allow it to focus. Viewing a clockface the astigmatic lens sees some of the lines as curving. It is not altered by the EB position or focus point *MT p7*. Assessed using a slit lamp which demonstrates the irregularity of the lens's curves.

Astrocyte supportive glial cell of the ON & CNS which protects and maintains strong N activity. Their processes form part of the BBB, by forming additional protection around the BVs and the N fibres. There are 2 main forms - the fibrous astrocyte (f) & the protoplasmic astrocyte (p).

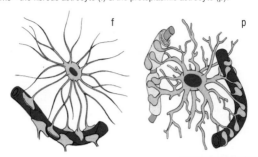

Atheroma fatty deposits on the inside of the arteries / arterioles – may impede or disrupt BF & make the arteriole wall stiffer & thicker

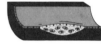

Atopic associated with allergies & over response of Abs *wrt eyes* atopic conjunctivitis AKA allergic conjunctivitis *(n Atopia)*

Atresia failure of the development of a tube or duct e.g. the tear duct in the eye

Atrophy degeneration/wasting of cells/structures due to lack of nutrition or use

Axis *wrt eye* the meridian specifying the orientation of a the cylindrical lens *adj axial pl axes see also Fick's axes*

Axial myopia myopia due to the lengthening of the EB *see also Myopia*

B

Background diabetic retinopathy (BDR) AKA non-proliferative retinopathy retinal changes include: microaneuysms, "dot & blot" Hgs, hard exudates, dilation of retinal BVs but NOT neovascularization ≠ **proliferative retinopathy**

Bacterial conjunctivitis If of the conjunctiva characterized by mucopurulent discharge, redness of the eye & a feeling of grittiness *see also Conjunctivitis*

"Bag" AKA capsular bag slang term for the capsule of the lens left behind after the removal of the cataract

Bandage lens soft CL w/o any RP, used protect a damaged cornea

Bare sclera the exposed sclera after attaching the conjunctiva to the sclera directly, subsequent to EOM surgery

Barkan's membrane a membrane found above the trabecular meshwork of the ant. chamber, which blocks drainage of the AH causing congenital glaucoma

Basal cell carcinoma (BCC) slow growing Tm of the epi. with a pearly raised edge & develops central ulceration with ↑ size *wrt eyes* commonest malignancy of the ELs

Basal Iridectomy *see Iridectomy*

Basal secretion test measurement of the basal tearing rate in the eye by placing filter paper strips in the EL conjunctival fornix *part of the Schirmer test*

Basal tearing secretion of fluid by the lacrimal system (mainly the small accessory glds of the ELs) which maintains the eye's tear film

Basement membrane (BM) an acellular mucopolysaccharide layer ~0.05mm (2) found underneath any epithelium or endothelium (1). Nutrients

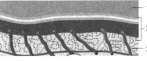

diffuse across this platform to these avascular layers. The BM is necessary for epi. migration & healing, connecting the epi. with the CT (3) underneath.

Battle's sign a bruise found in the mastoid area (behind the ears) suggesting there may be a basal skull #

"Bear tracks" AKA congenital grouped pigmentation an anatomical variant where areas of hyperplastic RPE are seen, resembling footprints

Bedewing (beh-DEW-ing) AKA corneal bedewing AKA Sattler's veil swelling & cloudiness of the supf. corneal layers due to irritation of CLs or ↑ IOP

Bell's palsy AKA facial palsy resulting from ly to the Facial N = CN VII & paralysis of facial muscles on one side, ss include: facial droop, upper EL ptosis (1) & lower EL ectropion (2), and drying of the cornea & sclera due to poor EL closure *see also Ectropion*

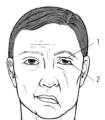

Bell's phenomenon upward & outward EB deviation with EL closure

Benedikt's syndrome paralysis of EOM in one eye (from CN III) with assoc. contralateral arm tremor

Bonign (buh-NĪN) an uncontrolled but non-metastasizing growth (≠ **malignant**)

Benign essential blepharospasm uncontrolled blinking from muscle spasm of Orbicularis Oculi m often assoc. with uncontrolled spasms of the face & neck

Benson's sign *see Asteroid hyalosis*

Beri Beri syndrome resulting from thiamine (Vita B1) deficiency ss-bacterial conjunctivitis, Ins on the ELs & if severe ON degeneration & amblyopia

Berlin's oedema *see Commotio retine*

Bicanthal plane the transverse plane linking both canthi; dividing the face into the upper & midface regions *see also Canthus*

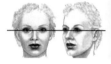

Bick's procedure shortening of the lower EL used to correct ectropion

Biconcave / Biconvex lenses double curved lenses as concave or convex

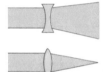

Bielschowsky head tilt test AKA Head Tilt test the head is tilted from R to L in order to determine where the true weakness of the EOMs lies in the hypertropia. *see Head Tilt Test*

Bielschowsky-Lutz-Cogan syndrome *see internuclear ophthalmoplegia*

Bietti's marginal crystalline dystrophy crystalline deposits in the corneal periphery assoc. with retinal pigmentation

Bifocals AKA Bifocal Lenses or Contact lenses corrective lenses with 2 different prescriptions generally the upper lens will correct far sightedness & the lower, near-sightedness & they may be *lined* with obvious differences b/n the 2 different strengths or *progressive* with graduation b/n the 2 strengths

Birefringence separation of light in 2 planes of polarization with a 90° separation

Binocular vision the combination of the 2 images formed from the 2 eyes transformed into a single clear image - with depth perception

Biogenesis the development or formation of ...e.g. biogenesis of an organelle may result from the fusion of several components ± their further modification

Biomicroscope *see Slit lamp*

Blepharitis If on the EL, including local Ifs such as styes

blepharo (BLEF-ar-oh) pertaining to the eyelid

Blepharoclonus abnormally long closure phase in blinking - exaggerated blinking

Brightness acuity test AKA Glare test determination of the effect on VA of a bright light straight at the eye - a determination of the extent of cataract impairment

Brown's syndrome AKA SO Sheath syndrome sheath of the SO cannot relax when looking up & it appears as a palsy of the IO - part of the restrictive syndromes

Brucke's muscle longitudinal fibres of the ciliary muscle to control the trabecular meshwork spacing & hence the IOP

Brückner test (BROOK-ner) used to detect strabismus - part of the **Red Reflex**, shining a light into the eyes illicts a red glare - the brighter is from the deviating eye (should be even)

Bruit (BROO-ee) sound hear over turbulent flow in an artery assoc. with abnormal arteries *wrt eye* - a bruit over the carotid a can be a sign of carotid cavernous sinus fistula, orbital or intracranial Tms

Brunescent cataract brown coloured cataract

Brushfield spots brown spots on the iris *see also Spots*

Busacca nodules AKA Koeppe nodules clumps of If cells on the front surface & pupillary border of the iris assoc. with uveitis

bucco (buko) pertaining to the cheek

Bulb of the eye, is the eyeball **AKA Globe**

Bulbar sheath AKA Fascia bulbi

Buphthalmos large EB in infantile glaucoma *see also Brakan's membrane*

C

Campimeter instrument for testing the VFs - detects loss or inattention in the peripheral fields

Calcarine fissure midline sulcus (groove) in the occipital lobe of the brain separating the upper & lower 1/2s.

Canal tunnel/ extended foramen as in the carotid canal at the base of the skull *adj canular*

Canal of Schlemm AKA Sinus Venosus Sclerae a modified circular venous structure (4) at the base of the cornea, in the anterior chamber (7) which drains the AH to the aqueous veins (2) via the scleral venous plexi (1) through large collecting channels (3), or directly via the conjunctival veins (5). It also drains the scleral arteries (6).

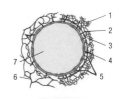

Canaliculus (CAN-al-ik-EW-lus) AKA Canicule (CAN -ik-kewl) small canal (*in the eye* – often describes the tear ducts of the ELs)

Candela measurement of luminosity based on the standard light bulb

Candida Albicans yeast-like fungus infects the eye & adnexae particularly in the immunodepressed patient

Candlewax drippings descriptive term for waxy exudates in the VB & retinal surface assoc. with sarcoidosis

Cannula small tube-like device for injecting or extracting air or fluids

Canthus (KAN-thus) AKA Palpebral commissure AKA the corner of the eye either corner of the eye where the eyelids meet, laterally (1) or medially (2), also described as the angle(s) / end(s) of the palpebral fissure *pl canthi*

Canthotomy generally refers to the cutting of the lateral commissure to widen the palpebral fissure

Capillary smallest BV in the system endothelial lining w/o a muscle layer or adventitia

Capillary dropout loss of retinal capillaries due to vascular disease e.g. DM, TIA or venous occlusion also seen in hypertension as it manifests in the eye

Capsule *wrt eye* elastic bag enveloping the crystalline lens, with properties of the BM. It is the thickest BM in the body, varying from 4μm posteriorly to 21μm anteriorly.

Capsulectomy removal of part or all of the lens capsule

Capsular bag *see Bag*

Capsulorhexis AKA Capsulotomy opening of the capsule for the removal of the lens

Carcinoma malignant Tm of epithelial derived T. Three common types:

> **Basal cell carcinoma (BCC),** *see Basal cell carcinoma*
>
> **Sebaceous gld Tm** *see Sebaceous glds*
>
> **Squamous cell carcinoma (SCC)** *see Squamous cell carcinoma*

Cardinal fields *see Diagnostic fields of gaze*

Caruncle (KAR-un-kul) *(Gk caruncula = wart)* wart fleshy growth *wrt eye* the small fleshy growth at the medial canthus (1) covering the LA *see Canthus, Lacrimal caruncle Plica semilunaris (2)*

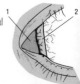

Cataract (KAT-ar-akt) *(Gk clouding)* opacity of the lens in the eye which may cause blurring of vision &/or diplopia by diffusing the incident light & preventing clear focus on the retina. This opacity may occur in the centre - **nuclear**, under the capsule **subcapsular** or in the cortex **cortical** *see also MT p244*

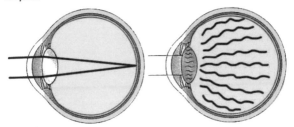

Cations positively charged atoms or radicals e.g. NAD^+, Na^+, H^+, Ca^{++}

Caput / Kaput the head or of a head, ***adj.- capitate = having a head (c.f. decapitate)***

Capitus AS Capitis pertaining to the Head

Cavity an open area or sinus w/n a bone or formed by two or more bones ***(adj. cavernous)***, may be used interchangeably with fossa. Cavity tends to be more enclosed fossa a shallower bowl like space (cf Orbital fossa-AKA Orbital cavity).

"Cell & Flare" presence of WBCs & proteins in the ant chamber *see also **Aqueous flare***

Central fixation AKA Fixation coordination of the EOM & the IOM so that the eyes converge and focus on the same image on their fovea

Central foveal reflex the sharply defined reflection from the fundus of the eye when a light is shone directly onto the fovea, if this is distorted it is an early sign of a cataract *see Macula*

Central retinal artery occlusion (CRAO) sudden permanent VL with retinal changes: opaque inner layers, cherry red macula & thin retinal arteries in the acute stages. These fade over time

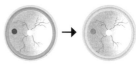

Central retinal vein occlusion (CRVO) AKA Retinal apoplexy AKA Haemorrhagic retinopathy severe ↓ VA & developing VL, retinal changes include; engorged veins, intraretinal Hgs (1), papilloedema (2), optic cupping & retinal thickening (3) & ↑ IOP

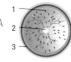

Central scotoma AKA Blind spot a physiological defect in the temporal VF at the point of the ON entry, no more than 5^n

Central vision images of the macular region

Centre of Rotation a point w/n the EB about which it rotates for movement - the meeting point of Fick's axes

Centrocecal scotoma loss of central vision including the fixation point & blind spot - indicative of toxic damage to the ON *see also Scotoma*

cephalo- pertaining to the head

cervico- pertaining to the neck

Cerebellopontine tumour tumour b/n the Pons & Cerebellum involving CNs V-VIII, hence impaired hearing & oscillating eye movements & blepharospasm & loss of the corneal reflex

Chalcosis (KAL-koh-sis) deposits of copper in the iris & lens - causes a sunflower cataract

Chandler's syndrome AKA Essential Iris atrophy holes form in the iris & the pupil is distorted assoc with severe glaucoma

Chalazion (KUL-ayz-ee-on) AKA Hordeolum chronic granulomatous If of a meibomian gland DD sebaceous gld Tm *pl chalazia*

Check ligament a fibrous T attachment which "checks" the eye from OA in both abduction & adduction

Cheiroscope device used to reverse visual suppression in the deviated eye - one eye views an image & the other eye looks as it is redrawn - visual input from both eyes is needed to complete this task

Chemosis (KEEM-oh sis) conjunctival oedema

Cherry red spot apparent colour change of the fovea from an opacification of the surrounding thicker retinal layers (as in metabolic storage diseases), leaving the thinner more transparent macular region to appear red due to the choroid BVs. It is also seen in the acute stage of CRAO, bc of the surrounding infarcted retinal arteries *see Central retinal artery occlusion*

Chiasm AKA Chiasma AKA Optic Chiasma (KĪ-azm) the point at which the nasal 1/2 the ON fibres from each eye cross to the other side - note its close relation to the stalk of pituitary gland (1), mamillary bodies (2) & internal carotid vessels (3) & other vessels of the circle of Willis (4). Pressure or changes to any of these structures will affect the VP.

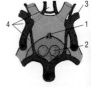

Chiasmal suppression syndrome pressure from above &/or below result in temporal VFD

Chlamydia trachomatis MO which causes trachoma - leading cause of blindness *see also Trachoma, Trichiasis*

Choriocapillaris the inner capillary layer (1) of the choroid, derived from its arterioles (2a) & venules (2v), which abuts the Bruch's membrane (2) & is responsible for the BS of the RPE (3). Drusen are found in b/n these capillary pillars (4).

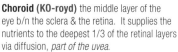

Choroid (KO-royd) the middle layer of the eye b/n the sclera & the retina. It supplies the nutrients to the deepest 1/3 of the retinal layers via diffusion, *part of the uvea.*

Choroid detachment AKA Choroidalis separation of the choroid from the sclera due to fluid leakage of the choroidal BVs 2° to ly & rapid ↓ IOP

Choroidal folds folds seen in the back of the eye due to localized IOP changes from a localized source e.g. a tumour

Choroidal neovascularization (CNV) abnormal BVs in choroid which are associated with wet macular degeneration

Chromphobe adenoma tumour of the pituitary which places P on the chiasm; may present as temporal VFDs

Chronic of long standing

Cicatrix (SIK-ar-triks) AKA scar *adj cicatricial* - caused by or related to a scar

Cilium / Cilia AKA eyelash/es *(in the eye)*

Ciliary body(CB) the structure behind the iris: produces the AH, alters the state of the lens & facilitates the drainage of the ant. chamber

Ciliary flush AKA Ciliary injection AKA Ciliary hyperaemia external eye redness caused by congestion of the deep BVs surrounding the limbus, assoc. with corneal If, iritis &/or acute angle glaucoma

Ciliary sulcus groove in the post. chamber b/n CB & the iris root - may be used as a stabilizing point in lens surgery

Cilioretinal artery variant found in 15% where some of the BS to the macula comes from a branch of the ciliary or choroidal BVs

Ciliospinal reflex pupil dilatation in response to painful stimuli, partic at the back of the neck

Clinical trial a research study which monitors patient progress as they proceed with new medication &/or Tx which is not necessarily available to the public

Circle of Zinn AKA Common tendinous AKA Annular tendon AKA Annulus of Zinn

Cloquet's canal AKA Retrolental tract AKA Hyaloid canal the central portion of the VB (1) following the path of the embryonic hyaloids BVs; it attaches to the posterior surface of the lens to the OD and is surrounded by 2 other more peripheral zones of the VB

Coloboma (KO-loh-boh-mar) *(Gk defect)* a congenital defect causing an incomplete growth in one or more of the features of the eye: iris, lens &/or retina. The effect on the person's vision is varied

Colour blindness AKA Colour deficiency a defect in visual perception of colour *see also Blindness*

Common Tendinous Ring *see Annulus of Zinn*

Commotio Retinae (KUM-oh-SHEE-oh RET-in-ee) AKA Berlin's oedema swollen white "bruised retina" from direct blunt trauma, VL, poor Px if this is in macula region

Compact bone = Cortical bone = Dense bone bone found in the shafts & on external bone surfaces highly structured in concentric circles or Haversian systems constantly changing & remodeling depending upon the lines of force, often enclosing the lighter trabecular bone.

Concave lens AKA divergent AKA minus AKA negative AKA reducing lens a lens which causes the light rays to diverge used to correct myopia or nearsightedness *see also Convex*

Concha (KONG-ku) a shell shaped bone as in the ear or nose *(pl. conchae adj. chonchoid)* old term for this turbinate.

Cones specialized cells in the retina which are sensitive to colour & light in the daylight - they are found throughout the retina but densest in the macular region *see also Rods*

Confocal microscope HP version of the slit lamp biomicroscope used to see the corneal details in corneal Ins

Conjugate movement *see Gaze movement*

Conjunctival chalasis AKA Conjunctivochalasis loose bulbar conjunctiva which intereferes with EL closure

Conjunctival follicles present in forms of conjunctivitis - formed from lymphoid T

© A. L. Neil

Congruous field defects VFD similar in both eyes generally due to brain lesions in the occipital lobes or post. optic radiation

Conical cornea see Keratoconus

Conjunctivitis If of the conjunctiva with discharge & capillary injection in the fornix - the cornea & pupil are unaffected
Types described by their morphology include: **bacterial, contact (allergic), dermato-** involving the adjacent skin & adnexae of the eye, **follicular, giant papillary** assoc. with the wearing of CLs, **haemorrhagic** assoc. with adenovirus, **phlyctenular** reactive If to the bacterial Ag at the limbus, **vernal (allergic) & viral see also follicle & papilla see also MT p250**

Consensual light reflex contraction of one pupil when the other is exposed to light *see also Swinging Light Reflex, Marcus Gunn pupil*

Constrictor to squeeze - generally referring to a muscle's action where it decreases the size of an opening (cf Papillary Constrictor - the muscle which ↓ the pupillary diameter)

Contact arc distance b/n an EOM initial contact with the sclera & its insertion into the EB related to tendon length and insertion point *see also Spiral of Tillaux*

Contact lenses (CL) literally lenses which make contact with the eye there are several types - hard, soft & scleral

contra- opposite of /on the opposite side to

Contraindicative refers to Tx which will worsen the condition

Contralateral synergists AKA Yoke muscles 6 pairs of EOM which move the eyes in the same direction *see also Yoke muscles*

Contusion AKA Bruise blunt ly which does not break the skin or wall of the EB

Convergence (≠ Divergence) the process of directing the visual axes to a near point
adj convergent

Types: **accommodative** - to focus on a single near object
> **fusional** - to maintain a single image in a moving object or with an esophoria
> **tonic** - change from sleep to waking
> **voluntary** - the maximal convergence possible irrespective of focus

This may be assisted with corrective lenses *see also Concave, Convex & Lenses*

Convergent insufficiency cannot converge enough to focus on a single image *see also Diplopia, Double vision, Asthenopia*

Convergent spasm inward eye deviation often hysterical *see Esotropia*

Convex lens AKA convergent AKA magnifying AKA plus lens a lens which causes the light rays to converge, used to correct hyperopia &/or presbyopia and focus on near objects *see also Concave*

Copper wiring colour of an opacified retinal arteriolar walls assoc with BP ↑ & atherosclerosis *see also Silver wiring (a more advance form)*

Corectopia displacement of the pupil from its normal position

Coreoplasty surgery to the pupil usually to dilate it *see pupillomydriasis*

Corneal abrasion any scratching of the cornea due to a FB – may be a deep erosion on the surface (1) or due to a FB trapped under the EL leaving vertical scratches as the EL blinks (2) Fluorescein drops onto the surface will detect any corneal defect (3)

Corneal decomposition AKA Corneal dystrophy AKA endothelial dystrophy AKA Fuch's dystrophy failure of the endothelium to seal the inner corneal surface causes thickening of the cornea + clouding & lack of transparency with white hyaline deposits & blisters on the cornea (guttata); often hereditary assoc. with VA ↓ & pain

Corneal dellen AKA Dellen localized corneal thinning generally at the limbus

Corneal ectasia AKA Keratoectasia *see Keratoconus*

Corneal hydrops sudden accumulation of fluid w/n the cornea resulting in clouded vision *see also Keratoconus*

Corneal melts *see Keratolysis*

Corneal ulcer defect in the epithelium

>**Mooren's** painful loss of epithelium due to chronic If usually near the limbus ↑ with age
>**Terrien's** thinning of the of the cornea near the limbus with fatty deposits & neovascularization causes - ↑ astigmatism, ± leakage of ant. chamber fluid & perforation then phthsis

Corneoconjunctival intraepithelial neoplasia AKA Bowen's disease progressive but slow growing malignancy at the limbus characterized by nodules confined to the epithelium - a precursor to SCC assoc with sun exposure

Corneal adenoma AKA Fuch's adenoma small white nodule of non-pigmented epithelium in the CB pars plicata

Corona a crown. *adj.- coronary, coronoid or coronal;* hence a coronal plane is parallel to the main arch of a crown which passes from ear to ear *(c.f. coronal suture).*

© A. L. Neil

Cortex outer rim or layer *wrt eyes* thc jcllylikc ccntre of the lens containing millions of lens films b/n the inner hard nucleus and outer elastic capsule / *wrt brain* **AKA Grey Matter** outer neuronal layer of the brain

Cortical blindness AKA Cerebral blindness blindness due to damage to the BS of the occipital lobe Brodman's area 17; the retina is normal but the visually evoked electrical response is significantly reduced

Cotton wool spots AKA Soft exudates "fluffy " white deposits on the retina due to ischaemia of the retinal BVs because of occlusion of the retinal as – a progression of the "silver wiring" seen in the retina. They disappear after weeks but leave permanent VL

Couching archaic term for displacement of the lens by blunt ly to the eye

Cover tests various test where one eye is covered & the other watched for changes in EB movement - will uncover a latent eye misalignment / deviation *see also Tropias, Trophias*

COWS mnemonic for the test used to detect balance of the inner ear & eye movement; placing **C**old water in the ear causes rhythmic oscillations to the **O**pposite side, but placing **W**arm water will cause these to occur to the **S**ame side

Cranial arteritis AKA Giant cell arteritis AKA Temporal arteritis If of the arteries which supply the head & eyes assoc with severe headaches, fever, wgt loss, stroke, heart attack *wrt eyes*: there may be sudden VL, ON If, diplopia & ptosis, if the central BVs are involved

Cranium the cranium of the skull comprises all of the bones of the skull except for the mandible *adj cranial* e.g. Cranial Nerves are those which leave the cranium not the spinal cord

Crawford's tubes tubes placed in the nasolacrimal duct to keep it patent – may remain in place for months

Crescent (myopic) semilunar structure seen just temporal of the OD in high myopes (severely myopic EBs)

Crest prominent sharp thin ridge of bone formed by the attachment of muscles particularly powerful ones e.g. Temporalis/Sagittal crest

Cribiform / Ethmoid a sieve or bone with small sieve-like holes.

Cribiform ligament the ligament seen at the entrance of ON into the retina

Cricoid (KRĬ-koyd) a ring

-crine to secrete

Cross-eye(d) *see Strabismus*

Cryotherapy Tx using cold to freezing temperatures. One of the rationales for this is that it slows the T metabolism and so allows it to be anoxic for longer periods w/o damage - another is that it ↓ P & BF in the region

Crystalline lens AKA Lens the flexible transparent globular body directly behind the iris which focuses the incident light to the retina - generally in macular region. If this clear lens develops an opacity, it is called a cataract.

Cul-de-sac AKA conjunctival sac AKA fornix AKA palpebral fornix empty sac b/n EB & EL allows the eye to move freely and stops CLs from moving behind the eye

Cup-to-Disc ratio numerical expression indicating the percentage of OD occupied by the optic cup - used to measure the progression of glaucoma *see Optic cupping*

Cupping the indentation in the OD that often occurs in glaucoma & other diseases states where IOP ↑ *see Optic Cupping*

Cutaneous Horn a keratinous skin growth generally benign but maybe pre-cancerous frequently found on the face and hands - *wrt eye* it is found on the edge of the EL

Cutus (KEW-tis) skin - *adj cutaneous* includes the epidermis + dermis

Cyclectomy AKA iridiocycletomy removal of the CB and its assoc. iridal segment

Cyclitic membrane (si-KLIH-tik) membrane of fibrous T & If cells that grows across the front surfaceof the VB - causing VL & shrinkage (phthsis) of the EB 2° to IO If

cyclo to do with the CB

Cycloablation destruction of part of the CB to ↓ aqueous fluid production performed by various means :- freezing, -cyclocryotherapy; surgery - cyclopexy

Cyclodialysis separation of CB from sclera - from blunt trauma or surgery to form a channel to allow for better drainage of the aqueous fluid

Cycloduction rotation of the CB around the centre of fixation - Fick's Y axis / torsion - hence it will point inward or outward (to the nose or to the temple) *see also Diagnostic fields of gaze & muscle movements MT p254*

Cyclophotocoagulation lazer ablation of parts of the CB

Cycloplegia paralysis of the CB

Cycloplegic adjective to describe a drug which relaxes the CB muscle - ciliaris via the PaNS and paralyzes accommodation

Cyclotropia EOM imbalance in which vertical axes of both eyes in the same direction *see also Torsion*

Cylindrical lens lens that produces a different RE in each meridian (axis) used for astigmatism ≠ concave or convex

Cyst (SIST) thin walled sac

Cystic oedema AKA cystoid macular oedema AKA Irvine-Gass syndrome retinal swelling or cyst formation in the macula, generally post-cataract surgery - settles in most cases in weeks

Cystotome instrument used to open the front of the capsule of the lens

D

dacro- to do with tears / lacrimal apparatus

Dacroadenitis If of the lacrimal gld - may occur post mumps

Dacryocystitis If of the tear ducts

Dacrocystocoele outpouching of the tear sac

Dacrocystorhinostomy surgical operation to refashion a tear duct from the lacrimal sac due to blocked nasolacrimal duct

Dacrostenosis narrowing of the tear duct

Dacryolith small stone in the tear duct

Dalen Fuch's nodules If cell clusters beneath the RPE assoc. with sympathetic ophthalmia

Dark adaptation AKA Scotopic vision AKA rod vision AKA mesopic vision ability & rapidity to adapt to low illumination generally to fully adapt takes 30 mins, but this slowed when there is an obstruction of the light pathway to the retina; while this is related to Night Blindness they may be separate entities *see also Night Blindness*

Decussation crossing e.g. Ns or light rays

Dehiscence breaking apart / down as in degenerative opening a wound previously healing

Dellen *see Corneal dellen*

Dendrite N processes which bring information to the neural cell body

Dendriform tree-like c.f. dendritic keratitis - which is a superficial corneal ulcer which is from the Herpes Simplex virus *see also Corneal ulcers, Keratitis*

Dens a tooth, denticulate having tooth-like projections *adj dental, dentate, dentine denticulate*

Densitometry AKA Reflective densltometry measuremcnt of various photopigments in the visual cells

Deosumvergence downward movement of one eye in relation to the other *see also eye movements*

Deosumversion `AKA Infraduction AKA Depression downward movement of both eyes from the straight ahead position

Depression a concavity on a surface *wrt eyes* - a downward movement of both eyes

Depressors EOMs which move the EB downwards (IR, SO)

Depth of field range/ distance in which an image is sharp

Depth Perception awareness of relative spatial location of objects
> **binocular AKA Stereopsis** 2 slightly different images are projected onto the retina

monocular geometric perception using clues of shadows, size and speed ***see also Parallax***

Dermatitis If of the skin - *wrt eyes* - affects the ELs & conjunctiva (dermo-conjunctivitis)

Dermatochalasis AKA Blepharochalasis excessive skin on the EL

Dermoid cyst AKA dermoid epibulbar dermoid Tm with skin elements generally found at the limbus or upper EL

Descemet's membrane AKA posterior limiting membrane similar to a BM in the cornea acellular layer supporting the corneal endothelium, and ending the extent of the stroma ***see also Basement membrane, Bowman's membrane, Bruch's membrane***

Desmosome site of local adhesion b/n cell membranes

Desquamated the shedding of keratinized layer of the skin

Detachment separation of layers from each other - particularly relevant in the eye as it is a series of interdependent layers

Types : **choroidal** - sep b/n choroid & sclera 2° to ly & leakage of fluid from the choroid causes ↓ IOP

CB - sep. of the CB from the sclera 2° to ruptures of the scleral spur causes a soft EB

Descemet's - post surgery - causes the cornea to swell become cloudy and soften

RPE - separation b/n RPE & Choroid as part of MD but if small may reverse w/o effect

post. viteous / vitreous - VB separates from the retina - may cause retinal tears &VL otherwise innocuous

retinal - separated from the RPE - due to a retinal tear is an emergency if there is to be no VL

serous - a general term for any detachment

Deturgesence ↓ swelling usually in the water content of the cornea

Deutan (DEW-tan) colour vision deficiency involving green (often difficulty in distinguishing b/n red & green) - deuteranomaly - milder form than deuteronopia

Deviation AKA Heterotropia AKA Squint AKA Strabismus AKA Tropia
eye misalignment due to EOM inbalance at all times ***see also Heterophoria, Phoria***

Primary deviation (1) - the non-deviated eye focuses in the primary gaze - both eyes receiving normal stimulation

Secondary deviation (2)
- the deviated eye focuses in
the primary gaze making the
non-deviated eye appear
deviated due in both cases to OA of the yoke EOMs as it takes an overstimulation to focus the deviated eye

1   2

dextro- to do with the right

Dextroversion movement of both eyes to the right

Diabetic Retinopathy a complication of DM, where the small BVs of the retina are blocked causing the growth of new fragile BVs which grow into the retina &/or the vitreous humour obscuring vision. If these BVs Hg this causes further loss of vision

Dialysis *wrt eyes* separation or a tearing of structures - (in medicine filtering of the fluids in the body)

Diaphoresis excessive sweating

Dichromatism absence of 1 or more colour perception

Diffuse widespread (**≠ Local**)

Digito-ocular reflex sensation of light in a blind eye - caused by rubbing the EB and activating the photoreceptors

Diktyoma (DIK-tee-oh-muh) Tm of the CB

Dilate to open or make bigger e.g. lacrimal punctum or pupil

Dilated Pinhole test AKA Pinhole test test for macula function in the presence of opacities such as corneal scarring or cataract - things appear clearer when looking through a small hole 0.5-2mm

Dilator muscle AKA Dilator Pupillae AKA Iris Dilator opens the pupil

Diopter (D) measure of RP of the lens or the degree of divergence or convergence
e.g.   2D - brings parallel rays of light to a focus 1/2 m
         3D - brings parallel rays of light to a focus of 1/3 m ***see also Prism Diopters***

Diplopia AKA Double vision - seeing one object as 2 – may occur in both eyes or one eye only where it is a sign of early cataract, irregular cornea including post laser Tx on the cornea

Types - **crossed/heteronymous** - due to outward deviation
- **uncrossed** - due to inward deviation
- **pathological** - due to mal-alignment of eyes - correctable until 8yo
- **physiological** - occurs when focusing on a near object - distant objects appear double

Disjunctive AKA Disconjunctive movement AKA Disjunctive version eyes move in the opposite direction to each other to focus, may occur in any of the axes *(≠ Conjunctive)*

Distal further away from the axial skeleton *(≠ Proximal)*
in dentistry = along the dental arch in posterior direction *(≠ Mesial)*

Distichiasis (dis-tik-Ĭ-uh-sis) 2X or more rows of ELs often irritates the cornea *see also Trichiasis*

Divergence ≠ Convergence the process of directing the visual axes away from a focal point - magnifying an image *adj. divergent*

Dk level measurement of the amount of oxygen transmission per unit thickness of a CL

Doll's Eye phenomenon AKA eye movement in the opposite direction of the head movement; keeps the eyes fixed on an object when the head is moved passively from side to side or up & down *see also Vestibule-ocular reflex*

Dominant eye eye used to do main tasks eg looking down a microscope etc. This eye will control the binocular vision and is associated with "handedness of the person" the person's dominant hand

Dorello's canal opening in the brain where CN VI enters the cavernous sinus, often covered over by the Trigeminal ganglion

Dorsal back – similar to posterior

Dorsal midbrain syndrome AKA Sylvian aqueduct syndrome AKA Tectal midbrain syndrome ↓ ability to move the eyes up & down due to lesions in the BStem near the vertical gaze centre – assoc with the inability to converge & ↓ papillary response to light *see also Argyll-Robertson pupil*

dorsi - back

'Dot & blot" haemorrhages tiny round Hgs in the retina usually OPL assoc with DM

"Dots" of ophthalmology *see Spots of Ophthalmology*

Double ring small OD surrounded by halo of reduced pigment and possibly an additional pigmented ring – assoc with ON dysplasia or hypoplasia

Double vision *see Diplopia*

Down's syndrome *wrt eyes* mongoloid slant (lower EL margins slant up towards the lateral Canthi, Brushfield's iris spots, cataracts, esotropia, myopia, blepharitis & keratoconus

Doyne's syndrome degenerative retinal disorder characterized by white Drusen in the macular area which increase

"Dragged" disc/ retina displaced T from their original site 2° to surgery, trauma &/or prematurity causes various forms of VL

Dropout *see Capillary dropout*

Druault's bundle group of fibrils in the developing VB replaced by the zonules to fix the position of the lens

Druse (DROOS) *pl Drusen* small yellow / white extracellular deposits appearing as glistening masses lodged in the Bruch's membrane, separating it from the RPE. They may be mistaken for chronic papilloedema. They ↑ with age normally, but if present in large numbers around the macular region are a sign of AMD, if not a contributing factor to it *see also Bruch's membrane*

Dry Eye syndrome AKA Keratitis sicca AKA keratoconjunctivitis sicca due to lack of a tear film or incorrect tear film ss gritty burning feeling in the eyes relieved temporality by artificial tears, assoc with other drying of Ts as in *Sjögen's syndrome*

Dyschromatopsia abnormal perception of colours in the VF or part of the VF associated with optic neuritis

Dyslexia difficulty in reading and interpreting letters w/o any abnormality in the VP

Dysmetria *see Ocular dysmetria*

E

"E-test" AKA E chart AKA Rolling Es chart of VA for the illiterate, foreign or children who cannot identify English letters but must instead are asked to recognize the orientation of an"E"

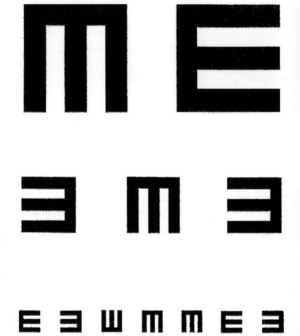

Eccentric fixation *see Deviation Fixation*

Ecchymosis (ek-EE-moh-sis) AKA bruise

Ectasia the dilatation of a tubular structure – used in ref to corneas

Ectropion turning out of the EL so that it exposes the EB as the ELs cannot completely close **see also Bell's palsy, Entropion, Trichiasis**

Elevation palsy paralysis of the upward gaze due to EOMs responsible (SR, IO)

Elschnig pearls cystic growths of the remnant capsular epithelium after cataract removal which resemble beads or bubbles **see also After-cataract**

Emmetropia absence of RE - normal focus **see also myopia & hyperopia**

Endolaser application of a laser into the globe

Endophthalmus sinking back into the socket of the EB generally due to loss of ocular fat (often present in older eyes) ≠ **Exophthalmus**

Endosomes membrane-bound body in the cell generally from ingested material and requiring further digestion – a progression in the path to lysosome differentiation **see also Lysosome, Vesicle**

Enophthalmia sunken EB

Endothelial dystrophy *wrt eyes see Corneal decomposition*

Entoptic phenomenon visual sensation arising from unusual stimulation of the retina eg P on the EB, the after image of a very bright light which will demonstrate the EB's own retinal BVs

Entropion turning in of the EL often causing irritation as the eyelashes rub against the sclera **see also Ectropion**

Enucleation complete removal of an EB commencing with: separation of the conjunctiva (1), division of the EOM (2), division of the ON (3), shelling of the globe & sewing together of the EOM (4)

Epicanthus AKA Eye fold AKA Palpebronasal fold congenital vertical skin fold that overlies the inner canthus seen most frequently in lower based nose bridges; present in the early foetus lost with nose definition **see also Canthus**

Epiphora (EPI-for-uh) tearing

Episcleritis If of the superficial conjunctival layer - characterized by the salmon-pink sclera, benign & self limiting **see also Scleritis**

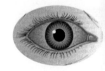

Epistaxis nosebleed

Epithelial basement membrane dystrophy AKA Cogan's microcystic dystrophy corneal epi BM forms cysts which expand with time distorting vision

Equator wrt eye AKA Anatomic equator line around the EB intersecting at right angles with the plane which divides the EB into front & back **see also Meridian**

Esophoria a tendency of the eyes to be convergent, which is not observed in normal sight but revealed in the covered eye - deviant eye circled, the normal eye does not change on covering

Esotropia a manifest inward deviation of one eye.

R esotropia when looking forward in the 1° position. If this is due to a paretic / weak EOM the disparity b/n the 2 eyes will alter on gaze changes, in this case a weakness of the RLR, causes this inward deviation of the R eye; hence gazing to the L will not have any disparity.

Evisceration removal of the contents of the eyeball

Exfoliated removal of the top layers of the skin

Exophoria a tendency for the eyes to be divergent - when both eyes are uncovered there will not appear to be any divergence - this is revealed when the weaker eye is covered when it is not bound by fusion - the normal eye's gaze does not change (Cover Test)

Exophthalmus bulging protrusive eye seen in Graves disease

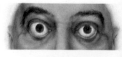

Exotropia a manifest outward deviation of one eye

R exotropia when looking forward in the 1° position. If this is due to a paretic / weak EOM the disparity b/n the 2 eyes will alter on gaze changes, in this case a weakness of the RMR, causes this outward deviation of the R eye; hence gazing to the R will not have any disparity.

Exudates secretions from cells onto an internal or external surface in the IR (≠ **infiltrate**)

Exudative macular degeneration AKA wet MD

extra- outside of

Eye chart (s) any device used to map or evaluate eye function including assessment of colour perception, contrast, VA, VF and other parameters

Eye colour AKA Iris

Eye socket AKA Orbital Fossa AKA Orbital Cavity

Eye drops topical medications for the surface of the EB

Eye strain *see Asthenopia*

Eyebrow areas of thick, delicate hairs above the eye that follow the shape of the lower margin of the brow ridges of the Frontal bone. Functions include: to prevent sweat & other debris from entering the eye, as a barrier against insects approaching the eye & as an aid to facial expressions. They are very mobile. Several muscles in the upper face can change their shape: Frontalis (5), Procerus(1), Corrugator (2), Orbicularis oculi has 2 portions the ocular (4o) & the palpebral (4p) which mainly affects the EL. The muscle inserts tightly on the medial side but more loosely (for mobility) on the lateral side via the lateral raphe (3).

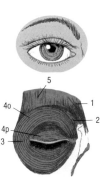

F

Facet (FASS-et) a face, a small bony surface (occlusal facet on the chewing surfaces of the teeth) seen in planar joints.

Far point the point at which the eye is focused when accommodation is completely relaxed

Facial N palsy *see Bell's palsy*

Farination small grey dot-like opacities on the corneal stroma near Descemet's membrane – incidental

Farnsworth tests tests with colour plates to evaluate patient's ability to discriminate b/n different hues

Far-sightedness AKA hyperopia

Fascia (FASH-ee-uh) face / CT generally in layers covering and connecting structures & organs to keep them in place

Fascia bulbi AKA Tenon's capsule AKA Bulbar sheath thin CT covering EB to the limbus – attaching EOM tendons to the FR

Fascia orbital collective term used for all the CT sheaths & tendons of the EB

Fascicule (FAS-ik-yewl) small bundle

Fast eye movements AKA Saccades AKA Rapid eye movements (REM) *see Saccades*

Febrile AKA feverish increased core body temperature generally due to In or IF (≠ **Afebrile**)

Fibril a small fibre or filament at least 10X smaller than the main type of fibrous structure and a smaller part of a larger structure as in myofibril

Fick's axes theoretical 3 axes X, Y, & Z through the centre of the EB and through which all the movements are measured *see also MT Movements of the Eye p194*

Field of vision the entire area that can be seen w/o shifting gaze - generally judged from the primary gaze

Fibre AS fiber *see also Filament* a rope or long strand of material - may have multiple subfibres or filaments in its makeup or appear as a single unit in biology there are 4 main types - the collagens; the elastins, the fibrillins & the fibronectins, but the most important by far is the collagen group *adj. fibrillar*

Filament *see also microfilament* a single thread or strand which may be thick or thin but is not made up of obvious multiple units as may be the case in a fibre

Fish-mouth tear a retinal tear opened by P on the overlying sclera

Fissure (FISH-er) a narrow slit or gap from cleft.

Fixation the act of fixing the 2 eyes on the one image - usually this is on the fovea (central fixation) but it may be more lateral with training in MD – eccentric fixation

Fixed dilated pupil *see Blown pupil*

Flap tongue or disc-shaped section of T dissected at 2-3 sides so it may be moved and reattached

Flare the bright light reflection of the healthy cornea (not the same as; aqueous flare AKA Tyndall effect)

Flashers AKA Lightning streaks sensation of light due to mechanical stimulation of the retina from newly formed : retinal tear, tugging on the VB, bumping or moving of the retina – possible detachment also a symptom of migraines

Flecked retina syndrome several retinal diseases in which white/yellow flecks appear on the retina, generally incidental

Flexure a fixed bend generally due to a tether by lig. or mesentery to the peritoneal wall as in the Hepatic flexure of the LI

Floaters AKA Muscae volintantes AKA Mouches volantes "objects" that appear to float across the eye - opacities &/or their shadows in the VB from precipitation of the vitreous gel into solid material. They may obscure vision, particularly when looked at on a plain light background, e.g. the sky. Contributing factors include dehydration & age.

Fluorescein (FLER-uh seen) dark orange dye that fluoresces a yellow-green when illuminated with UV light. *wrt eye* - used in retinal angiography & to detect corneal irregularities & evaluate the fit of CLs & tear drainage by direct application
Common patterns include: **1 Abrasion patterns** due to: a = astigmatism, b = embedded FB, c = central due to CL pressure, d = CL insertion, e = EL
2 spotted patterns: a = arc, b = bubbles - due to epithelial lifting , c = EL FB, d = strippling e = punctate **& 3 others** which include a = central cloudiness due to central oedema, b = 3 & 9 o'clock staining with ill-fitting CLs or keratoconus

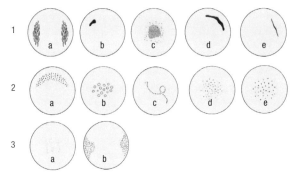

Focal distance the distance b/n the lens & the focal point

Focal Point (FP) the point at which focus is the sharpest on the retina

Focus the point at which the light rays are brought together to form an image, hence they do not form a point but an area when "out of focus"

Follicle *wrt eyes* small aggregate of lymphoid T (1) - similar to other lymphoid nodules, in the conjunctival layers under the conjunctival epithelium (2) seen in conjunctivitis *see also papilla*

Foramen (for-AY-men) a natural hole in a bone usually for the transmission of BVs &/or Ns. *(pl. foramina).*

Foreign body (FB) *wrt eyes* small particle or foreign object in the eye or its adnexae

Fornix corner, *wrt eye* the junction of the palpebral & bulbar conjunctiva *see also MT Conjunctiva p110*

Fossa a pit, depression, or concavity, on a bone, or formed from several bones as in temporomandibular fossa - shallower and more like a "bowl" than a cavity

Foveola small fovea – smaller area in the fovea (0.3mm) which is avascular & has only cone cells (it is that part of the macula which has the sharpest focus)

Free radicals unbound charged ions or molecules - highly reactive *see also Radicals*

Fuch's adenoma AKA Coronal adenoma is a peculiar mass which develops in the pars plicata of the CB.

Fuch's dystrophy *see corneal decomposition*

Fundus body *wrt eyes* the posterior portion of the EB visible via the pupil

Furrows grooves on the cornea – an indication of its thinning gen. pathological

Fusion combination of 2 images from the eyes into one

G

Gamma angle angle formed at the centre of the eye's rotation b/n optic axis & fixation axis

Ganglion group of N cells outside the CNS *pl. ganglia*
> **cervical** series of paired ganglia in the neck alongside the SC & internal carotid a
> **superior cervical** 1 pair in the neck containing sym N from cervical to thoracic which supply the eye & the orbit

Gasserian ganglion AKA Trigeminal ganglion

Gastric belly (as in the belly of a muscle)

Gaze movement AKA Conjugate movement AKA Subjunctive movement parallel movements of both eyes
> Left Gaze - looking left (RMR + LLR)
> Right Gaze - looking right (RLR + LMR) *see also Saccades*

Gaze palsy inability to make parallel movements, gen. indicative of brain lesions

Geniculate body AKA External geniculate body AKA Lateral geniculate body paired prominences on the sides of the midbrain (upper end of the Brain stem) where the optic tract fibres synapse with the optic radiation

Geniculo-calcarine tract AKA Optic Radiation visual N pathway b/n the lateral geniculate body & the calcarine fissure, containing the crossed nasal fibres & the uncrossed temporal fibres

Geographic *wrt eyes* a term used to describe a corneal ulcer, or other eye degenerative process which looks like a map & slowly expands

Geographic choroidalopathy bilateral progressive choroidal If which begins at the ON head (peripapillary) & slowly extends

Geometric axis AKA Optic axis line through the centres of curvature of the cornea & lens, which passes through the nodal point of the EB

Geometric Equator *see Equator*

Gerontoxon AKA Arcus Senilis

Ghost cells abnormal RBCs that can clog the trabecular meshwork with ↑ IOP

Ghost vessels remnants of BVs in cornea remaining after an If process when new BVs were induced to grow into the normally avascular

Giant cell arteritis *see Cranial arteritis*

Giant papillae small flattish elevations on the palpebral conjunctiva "cobblestones" each containing a tuft of BVs found in allergic & CL conjunctivitis

Giant tear retinal tear of at least 90° (1 quadrant) near the ora serrata or equatorial zone of lattice degeneration, which leads to retinal detachment

Giemsa stain used on conjunctival / corneal smears to identify different WBCs

Gierke's disease hepato-renal glycogenesis , inability to store glycogen - cloudy edges of the cornea

Glabella forehead b/n the eyebrows

Gland epithelial cells which secrete material that has an effect on other cells

Glare undesirable sensation produced by a brightness more intense than the eye's adaptation

    veiled glare a glare coming from a reflected surface

Glaucoma (GLOR-koh-muh) disease characterized by OD cupping & VF loss generally due to progressive ↑ IOP. If chronic, this may be silent, so the patient is unaware of the VL until, it is quite significant. Acute glaucoma is an emergency - due to the sudden blockage of AH drainage (1) which suddenly raises IOP (2), causing corneal cloudiness (3) & acute scleral injection (4) *see MT p260*

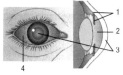

Glaucomatocyclitic crisis 2° glaucoma to uveal If -generally in 1 eye: ss corneal swelling leads to ↓ flow open anterior chamber angle

Glia (GLEE-uh) AKA Neuroglia supporting cells of the CNS, much like the CT of the body *see also Astrocytes*

Glioma (GLĪ-om-uh) tumour of the glia – or supportive cells in the CNS
    Optic Nerve Glioma slow growing Tm of the ON congenital ss large EB with EB protrusion

Globe AKA Eyeball (EB) AKA Orb

Glycan a sugar

Glycosylation attachment of 1 or more sugars to a molecule

Goblet cells large superficial mucous glands in the conjunctiva which secrete mucin, a component of the tear film - absent or damaged in Dry eye syndrome

Gonioscope special lens used to examine the ant. chamber of the eye

Goniosynechiae AKA Peripheral anterior synechia abnormal adhesion binding the front surface of the peripheral iris to the back surface of the cornea - near the ant. chamber angle ↓ flow and ↑IOP - glaucoma

Gradenigo's syndrome CN VI palsy with unilateral headache ± CN VII may follow a middle ear In

Graft transfer of living T to a new site *wrt eye* this may be the cornea, lens
> **autograft** T used is from the same person to the same person
> **free graft** T which has no attached BS ususally skin or conjunctiva
> **homograft** T used is from one individual to another
> **patch graft** T used is different from the site's T and is used only as a filler to maintain the shape or P of the eye or EB

Granuloma (gran-ew-LOH-mah) dense collection of cells consisting of many If cell types. Assoc. with chronic If conditions including FBs

Granulomatous uveitis non-purulent chronic If of the retina wherein cells & protein are found in the ant. chamber, fatty deposits are in the back of the cornea, a ciliary flush, conjunctival BVs are dilated & the pupils are small & irregular

Graticule measuring device or scale in an eyepiece of a microscope or other optical device

Grave's disease AKA Thyroid eye disease (TED) AKA Ophthalmopathy *wrt eyes* excess Thyroid H causes: EL retraction, EL lag, corneal drying, eye bulging, EOM fibrosis & ON If
see also Exophthalmos

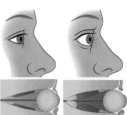

Grey AS Gray line AKA intramarginal sulcus line b/n the inner & outer EL margins, the conjunctiva & the skin eyelashes in front & the tarsal glds behind

Groove long pit or furrow

Gunn Pupil *see Afferent Pupillary defect*

Gunn's sign in hypertensive retinopathy "nicking" or narrowing of the venules both sides of the AV crossing due to the ↑ hardness of the a over the thin walled v

Guttata AKA "Corneal blisters" (GOO-tah-tah) white deposits on the inner surface of the cornea *see also Corneal decomposition*

H

H&E routine stain used in histology - demonstrating most organelles based on their affinity for acid & bases in contrasting blue (staining basophilic or acid substances) & pink (strongly staining bases or acidophilic substances) colours

Haab's striae breaks or tears in Descemet's membrane assoc. with congenital glaucoma

Haemangioma Tm composed of BVs may occur on the ELs or in the orbit

Haemorrhage (Hg) *wrt eyes*

> **choroidal** bleeding from ruptured choroidal BVs due to a sudden ↓ IOP
>
> **dot & blot** tiny round Hgs in the retina IPL assoc. with DM
>
> **expulsive** choroidal Hgs which may be extruded through the sclera
>
> **salmon patch** oval-shaped pale orange Hg in patients with sickle cell disease
>
> **subconjunctival** bright red blood overlying the scleral arising from coughing or spontaneously
>
> **subhyaloid** bleeding b/n VB & the retina surface layers
>
> **suprachoroid** outer layers of the choroid bleeding due to ↓ IOP or surgical procedures may proceed to expulsive Hg
>
> **viteous** blood in the VB from trauma, neovascularization, vitreous detachment &/or retinal tear

Haematoxylin ASA Hematoxylin *see H&E*

Haller's layer layer of large BVs in the outer choroid next to the sclera

Halo hazy ring seen around lights: assoc, with RE or optical defect

Hamartoma noncancerous Tm composed of T not fully differentiated in their development

Hamus a hook hence the term used for bones which "hook around other bones or where other structures are able to attach by hooking - hamulus = a small hook.

Haplopia a single image formed when corresponding points are stimulated on the retinas of each eye

Hard exudates deposits in the retina containing fat & protein caused by excessive vascular leakage of the retinal BVs

Harmonious abnormal retinal correspondence binocular adaptation of the retinas to long standing deviation so that a single binocular image is seen from the fovea of the non-deviating eye and the non-fovea image of the deviated eye ***see also unharmonious abnormal retinal correspondence, normal retinal correspondence***

Hasner's valve AKA Plica Lacrimalis MM fold at the lower end of the nasolacrimal duct, preventing air from entering the tear duct when the nose is blown

Haze diffuse scattering of light ↓ VA

> **aerial** atmospheric conditions which result in a blue haze surrounding distant objects
>
> **corneal** defects on the corneal surface which scatter the light entering the EB
>
> **stromal** defects in the corneal stroma
>
> **sub-epithelial** defects in the corneal epithelium

Head tilt test moving the head from side to side to determine the extent & site of vertical gaze weakness. Tipping the head to the side of the paresis - the affected side shows the hypertropia - in this case the RSO is weak and tipping to the R demonstrates this whereas tipping to the L does not

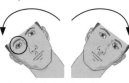

Helicoid spiral shaped

Hemianopia AKA Heminopsia blindness in ½ of the VF in 1 or 2 eyes

> **binasal** - VL in the nasal halves of each eyes VFs
>
> **bitemporal** - VL in the outer halves of both eyes
>
> **homonymous** - VL on the same side R or L of each eye caused by interruption or pressure at various levels of the VP

Hemidesmosome point attachment of the cm to the BM or another cell ***see also Desmosome***

Henle fibre layer structure in the foveal layer of the retina where the axon fibres in the OPL & IPL run obliquely

Henle's crypts & glands microscopic pockets with glands in the fornices along with the goblet cells which secrete mucous into the tear film

Hering's law innervation of 1 EOM will cause a corresponding innervation of the yoke muscle of the other eye so that gaze movement is possible ie RLR will cause LMR to be stimulated - hence in 2° deviation the deviated eye is more stimulated than in 1° deviation ***see also Deviation***

Hermeralopia normal vision in low light which decreases in bright light

Herpes simplex keratitis invasion of the cornea by the Herpes virus causes a typical dendritic pattern on the cornea with fluorescein drops

Heterochromia differences in eye colour b/n the 2 eyes of the one person

Heterophoria AKA Phoria tendency of the eyes to be misaligned – this is overcome by fusion – latent deviation , i.e. not obvious unless one eye is covered when the deviation will present itself ***see Exophoria, Endophoria***

Heterotopia AKA Ectopia misalignment of parts *wrt eye* refers to the dragged macula in retinopathy of prematurity & other retinal scars

Heteroptropia *see Strabismus*

Hippus exaggerated pulsating movements of the iris

Hirschberg test determines the relative position of an eye's deviation by testing the position of the corneal reflexes of both eyes

Histo spots small punched out holes usually w/o a pigmented border representing RPE & choroid scars assoc. ocular histoplasmosis

Holocrine secretions which involve the death of the cell with substance liberation

Homeostasis (HOH-me-oh-stay-sis) condition of cells in organs or tissues where loss of the units (cells usually) is equal to the formation of new units **A** - most disease states can be simplified to belong to an inequality b/n cell proliferation & loss either ↑ in loss as in atrophy **B** or ↑ in proliferation as in cancer **C**

Homograft AKA Allograft *see Graft*

Homologous corresponding in structure or appearance

Homonymous located on the same side c.f. homonymous hemianopia - VFD on the same side of both eyes *see also Scotoma*

Hordeolum (hor-DEE-oh-lum)
> **external AKA Stye (E)** acute pustular In of the Zeis glds in the EL or may affect the EL follicles
> **internal AKA Chalazion (I)** acute In of the Meibomian glds of the EL

Horizontal gaze centre AKA Pontine gaze centre region near the centre of the BStem at the level of the nucleus of CN VI believed to organize saccades

Horizontal meridian plane to divide the EB into upper & lower 1/2s

Horizontal raphe dividing line in the retina which separates the upper & lower N fibre layers, corresponds to a horizontal line on the nasal side of the VF

Horner's syndrome miosis, ptosis, & anhydrosis on the same side of the face caused by the paralysis of the sympathetic NS of the face

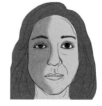

Horror fusionis unconscious avoidance of bifoveal fixation

Hruby lens (ROO-bee) attachment to the slit lamp which allows the examiner to observe the VB by neutralizing the power of the cornea (55D)

Hue aspect of a colour that gives it its name - corresponding to the wavelength of the light

Humour fluid

Hutchinson's pupil fixed dilated pupil that occurs due to the CN III compression often 2° to ↑ intracranial P

Hyaline masses *see Drusen*

Hyalitis AKA Vitritis If of the VB

Hyalocytes cells of the VB

Hyaloid a the main artery in the developing VB which supports the lens - later deteriorates to leave the VB clear & unobstructed

Hyaloid canal AKA Cloquet's canal AKA Retrolental tract the central portion of the VB following & containing remnants of the embryonic hyaloid BVs, hence it is devoid of collagen fibres.

Hyaloideo-capsular lig AKA Egger's line AKA Weiger's lig a weak line of adherence b/n the base of the VB & the post. surface of the lens

Hyaloid membrane membranous sheet on the vitreous surface
>**ant.** front surface layer - separates the VB from the ant. & post. chambers
>**post.** back surface layer firmly attached to the internal surface of the retina

Hydropic degeneration glycogen accumulation in the pigmented iris epithelium assoc. with DM

Hydrops AKA Corneal hydrops sudden influx of fluid to the cornea making it thicker & cloudy by changing the arrangement of the collagen lamellae

hyper- up / increased

Hyperaemia ↑ BF *wrt eye* **AKA Injection**

Hyperopia AKA Hypermetropia AKA farsightedness the focal point of the lens is behind the retina EB is too small
>**absolute** the amount of hyperopia after maximal accommodation
>**facultative = manifest**
>**high** when it is > 6D
>**latent** difference b/n manifest & total hyperopia
>**manifest** the amount of correction needed to give the patient full VA
>**total** entire amount of hyperopia in the eye

Hyperphoria tendency for upward gaze when the eye is covered, reversed when uncovered

Hypertelorism abnormally long distance b/n the 2 orbits, too widely spaced eyes leading to exotropia & assoc with mental retardation

Hypertropia AKA Manifest Vertical Strabismus upward deviation of one or both eyes, note the strabismus is named after the higher eye, even if this eye is used for fixation e.g. this is R hypertropia

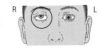

Hyphaema AS Hyphema (HĬ-feem-uh) B in the ant. chamber of the eye

hypo- below, lower, deficient

Hypopyon (HĬ-poh pĭ-on) pus in the anterior chamber of the eye

Hyposphagma (HĬ-poh-SFAG-muh) AKA subconjunctival haemorrhage AKA eye bruise bleeding in the fascial layer of the conjunctiva, due to increased P on the small BVs. The sclera appears as bright red, w/o corneal involvement. Like a bruise it is self limiting and may undergo similar colour changes before resolving in 1-2 weeks

Hypotony (hĭ-POH-toh-nee) low IOP related to uveitis & ly to the sclera, leads to retinal folds & BV engorgement

Hypotropia downward deviation of one eye *see also Eye movements*

Hysterical field tunnel vision - restricted VF due to hysteria may change during testing

Iatrogenic an adverse condition due to medical intervention

Idiopathic of unknown cause

Illusion a false or distorted sense of the environment due to a distorted sensory input rather than an hallucination which has no sensory input

Image visual impression of an object formed by a lens or a mirror
    false in diplopia the image from the deviating EB
    Purkinje the 4 reflected images back from the eye - from the front & rear surfaces of the cornea & lens -
    real image which can be focused on a screen from converging light rays
    true the image from the undeviated eye
    virtual back image from diverging rays cannot be focused on a screen

Implant material inserted into or grafted onto any Ts

> **intraocular** plastic lens that is surgically implanted to replace the natural lens
>
> **intrascleral** foreign material placed in/under the sclera to cover/heal gap in the seal
>
> **orbital** plastic or glass sphere placed in the socket under Tenon's capsule

Incise to cut w/o removal

Incisura a notch

Incycloduction AKA intorsion rotation of the EBs around the 12 o'clock meridian towards the nose while focusing

Infarct ischaemic cell death from lack of BS

Inferior under

Inferior longitudinal fasciculus N fibre tract through which visual fibres from the association areas in the occipital cortex pass to the temporal lobe

Inferior nasal a one of the 4 major br of the central retinal a - supplying the lower inner quadrant of the eye

Inferior temporal a one of the 4 major br of the central retinal a - supplying the lower outer quadrant of the eye

Inferonasal reference point below the EB & towards the nose

Infiltrate abnormal accumulation of cells & fluid in T *see also Exudate*

Inflammation / Inflammatory process (If) body's response to ly of any origin - 5 cardinal signs - dolor (pain), rubor (redness), calor (heat) tumour (swelling) & loss of function

Infraduction *see Deosumversion*

Infranuclear pathway N fibre bundles from a CN's nucleus to its site of action eg the eye

Inhibitional palsy of contralateral agonist longstanding EOM weakness - the weak muscle allows its direct antagonist to become OA hence the yoke muscle's contralateral antagonist in the other eye appears weak, hence RSO weakness is perceived as LSP weakness

Injection *wrt eye* T swelling assoc. with dilatation of the assoc BVs *see also Hyperaemia*

Inner retina retinal layers nearest the VB

Inner segment *wrt rods & cones* part of the cells which contain an ellipsoid portion of the mitochondria & myoid part of the GA

Inspissated refers to a secretion which has dried out

inter- between

Intercanthal distance distance b/n the R & L inner canthi

Interocular distance b/n eyes

Intermuscular AKA Muscle sheath CT sheath separating different muscle groups

Interpupillary distance distance b/n the R & L pupils - used for construction of glasses

Intercalated - e.g. intercalated discs or ducts inserted b/n other structures

Internuclear ophthalmoplegia AKA Bielschowsky-Lutz-Cogan syndrome due to lesions in the BStem -ss ipsilateral eye limited adduction contralateral eye limited abduction focus normal + nystagmus in both eyes assoc. with multiple sclerosis

Intra- within

Intraconal space fat-filled compartment of the orbit w/n the muscle cone behind the EB containing the ON, rectus m, intermuscular membranes, motor & sensory Ns

Intracranial pressure fluid P inside the skull controlled by the flow of CSF - normally 150-200mm water

Intraepithelial epithelioma *see Bowen's disease*

Intraocular inside the eye

Introitus an orifice or point of entry to a cavity or space.

Intumescent cataract a lens that has swollen & enlarged in the process of becoming cloudy

Iodopsin the visual pigment of the cone cells sensitive to red, blue or green

Ipsilateral anatagonist AKA direct antagonist muscles in the eye which opposes the action of the main action of the eye movement

Ions - charged atoms *see also Free Radicals*

     - -ve charge - anions - generally non-metal

     +ve charge - cations generally metal

Iridocyclectomy (i-rid-OH-sï klek-toh-mee) removal of CB with attached iris

Iridology study of the iris and ant. of the eye as a means of diagnosing systemic disease

Iris *(Gk rainbow)* the coloured multilayered portion of the eye surrounding the pupil. Its root lies in the CB just under the limbus *(pl irides/ irises)*

Iris prolapse iris protrusion into the sclera or cornea often after blunt trauma or surgery

Iritis If of the iris, characterized by small slightly hazy pupil, circumcorneal capillary injection or ciliary flush w/o discharge, in the chronic phase keratic precipitates are visible on slit lamp examination & the flush is more localized

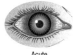
Acute

Chronic

Irvine-Gass syndrome *see Crystoid Macular Oedema*

Ischaemia (is-KEEM-ee yuh) death of a T due to oxygen deprivation *(adj ischaemic)*

Ishihara colour plates series of plates with coloured dots of similar shades but with variants in shades forming a number or shape – used to determine colour perception or its lack **AKA colour blindness**

Isometropia equal RF In both eyes (< 1/2 D difference)

Isopter boundary of the VF to a particular target – isopters of different colours allow differentiation of relative or absolute VF defects

-itis inflammation of

J

Jaeger test a chart of various lines of different widths to determine vision defects, particularly in near-sightedness

Johnson's syndrome *see Adherence syndromes*

Jones tests for evaluating the tear drainage in the eyes by placing blotting papers on the conjunctiva and timing the draining time for fluorescein into the nasolacrimal duct

K

K flattest part of the cornea important for the insertion of CLs

K-readings measurements of the corneal curvature - used to determine astigmatism

kerat- to do with the cornea

Keratic Precipitate (KP) accumulation of If cells on the post. cornea in uveitis

kp

Keratitis If of the cornea, often associated with intense pain

Keratitis sicca AKA Dry Eye Syndrome drying of the cornea due to exposure &/or reduced tear production *see also Dry Eye Syndrome*

Keratocoele protrusion of Descemet's membrane into the cornea to "plug" the ulcer

Keratoconus cone-shaped deformity of the cornea - the cornea thins which causes it to protrude forming a cone, may result from CL overuse

Keratocytes CT cells of the corneal stroma

Keratolysis AKA Corneal melt a sudden melting of the corneal supf. layers assoc. with keratitis & keratoconus

Keratomalacia softening of the cornea, associated with Vitamin A deficiency

Keratoplasty AKA Corneal graft

Köeppe nodule accumulation of If cells on the iris, observed in other If diseases involving the EB

Koplik's spots measle spots

Krause glands accessory tear glands located under the ELs in the fornices

L

Labia pertaining to lips *(adj labial)* may be oral or vulval lips

Labile easily changing

Labrador keratopathy *see Spheroid degeneration*

Lacerum something lacerated, mangled or torn e.g. foramen lacerum small sharp hole at the base of the skull often ripping tissue in trauma.

Lacquer cracks cracks seen in the Bruch's membrane indicative of the stretching of the EB in progressive myopia

Lacrima (LAK-rim-u) related to tears and tear drops. *(adj lacrimal)*

Lacrimal caruncle the small fleshy innermost structure in the medial canthus of the eye. It is a skin covered structure (1) which overlies the glds of the EL & the lacrimal duct and to which the fold of the bulbar conjunctiva attaches (2) before itself attaching to the sclera (3) *see also Canthus Plica semilunaris*

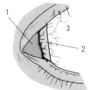

Lacuna *wrt eye* microscopic puddles in the retina *(pl Lacunae)*

Lagophthalmus (lag-OPF-thal-mus) inadequate EL closure when sleeping

Lambda (LAM-duh) from the Greek letter a capital 'L' and written as an inverted V. *(adj. lambdoid)* and used to name the point of connection between the 3 skull bones Occiput & the 2 Temporal bones. *wrt eyes* the Lambda angle is formed b/n the visual axis & the optic axis at the centre of the pupil

Lamella (LAH-mel-uh) - layer *(pl lamellae)*

Lamina a plate as in the lamina of the vertebra a plate of bone connecting the vertical and transverse spines *(pl. laminae)*

Lamina cribosa thin sieve-like portion of the sclera at the opening for the ON exit from tho oyo

Lamina dots holes in the lamina cribosa visible in the OD normal but more prominent with ON degeneration

Lamina papyracea (pah-pih-RAY-shee-uh) thinnest part of the orbit - lateral walls of the ethmoid sinuses, which are paper thin and form part of the medial orbital wall. Sinusitis may erode this wall and enter the orbit causing a severe cellulitis of the region including the EB.

Lamina propria (LP) proper layer, background T surrounding major specialized cell masses in an organ - often loose areolar T: a combination of CT, immune cells, BVs, lymphocytes & Ns

Lamina vitrea *see Bruch's membrane*

Latent hidden or masked

Lateral horn end of the LPS m in the upper EL attaching to the lat. palpebral lig. near the lat. canthus

Lateral medullary syndrome AKA Wallenberg syndrome common BStem stroke *wrt eyes* - dysmetria, Horner's syndrome, rotary nystagmus, skew deviations on the ipsilateral sides

Lateral Palpebral lig. strong fibrous band of T which anchors the upper & lower EL tarsal plates to the orbital tubercle on the Zygoma weaker than the medial palpebral lig

Lattice retinal degeneration retinal thinning with dense vitreous traction leading to retinal tears & detachment

Lazy eye *see Amblyopia, Strabismus*

Leber cells large macrophages seen in the conjunctivitis assoc. with trachoma

Left Gaze verticals EOM responsible for up & down eye movements when gazing left

(LIR, LSR, RIO, RSO)

Lens *see also Crystalline Lens* the solid structure in the eye which focuses the incident light contains capsule cortex and nucleus - the hardening of the nucleus is primarily responsible for presbyopia – also an external lens as in glasses which alter the RF of the eye

Legal blindness best-corrected VA of 6/60 (or 20/200) or less, reduction in the VF of 200 or less

Lesion localized abnormal change in a T due to Iy or disease

Leukocoria AKA Cat's eye reflex pale grey pupillary opening due to a cataract

Leukoma dense white opacity on a lens (smaller **macula**, more translucent **nebula**)

Levator to raise - generally in reference to the actions of muscles

Levoversion movement of both eyes to the L (≠ **dextroversion**)

Ligament a band of tissue which connects bones (articular ligaments) or viscera - organs (visceral ligaments). A ligament is a tie or a connection originally *sing. ligamentum pl. ligamenta* from ligate or to tie up generally composed of collagen fibres

Lid crease AKA Lid fold fold of upper EL when the eye is open

Lid lag AKA von Graefe sign slowing of the EL closure when looking down -ss of thyroid disease (Graves disease)

Ligand a small molecule, that forms a complex with a biomolecule to serve a biological purpose. Often used as a signal triggering molecule, binding to a protein which alters its shape to allow attachment of another protein often an H

Light adaptation adaptation of the eye to bright light **(≠ Dark adaptation)**

Light–near disassociation *see Argyll-Robertson pupil*

Light perception lowest level of light still detectable a test of this is used to determine extent of VP when VL is extensive

Light sensitivity AKA Photophobia (if severe)

Limbus AKA Corneoscleral junction *(Lt border) see Iris MT 178*

"Lines" of ophthalmology

> **Arlt's Line** - conjunctival scar in sulcus subtarsalis.
> **Ehrlich-Turck Line** - linear deposition of KPs in uveitis
> **Ferry's Line** - corneal epithelial iron line at the edge of filtering blebs.
> **Hudson-Stahil Line** - Horizontal corneal epithelial iron line at the inferior 1/3 of cornea due to aging.
> **Khodadoust Line** - corneal graft endo. rejection line composed of If cells.
> **Paton's Line** - circumferential retinal folds due to ON oedema.
> **Sampaoelesi line** - ↑ pigmentation anterior to Schwalbe's line in pseudoexfoliation syndrome.
> **Scheie's Line** - pigment on lens equator & post. capsule in pigment dispersion syndrome.
> **Schwalbe's Line** - Angle structure representing peripheral edge of Descemet's membrane.
> **Stockers Line** - corneal epithelial iron line at the edge of pterygium
> **White lines of Vogt** - sheathed or sclerosed BVs seen in lattice degeneration

Line of Fixation AKA Line of sight AKA Visual axis line b/n the object & the fovea in the eye

Linea (lin-EE-uh) a line as in the nuchal lines of the Occipitum

Lipaemia retinalis white retinal BVs due to high fat content in the B

Lipofuscin normal brown pigment seen in the skin and in the retina ↑ with age & some disease states

Lingual (ling-GEW-al) pertaining to the tongue

Lisch nodules raised pigmented nodules on the iris assoc. with neurofibromatosis

Listing's law as an eye moves from the primary position to an oblique position the amount of torsion is independent of the route to get there

Listing's plane plane in the eye passing through the equator *see also Fick's axes*

Lockwood's ligament lower thickened portion of fascia bulbi, fascial band under the eye formed by blending of sheaths of IO & IR; extends to the orbital walls, orbital septa & lower tarsus, forming a sling under the EB, loosening of this lig is associated with ectropion of the EL

Loops of Axenfeld AKA interscleral N loops loops of the long ciliary N to the ant. sclera appear as tiny dark spots of uveal T on the sclera near the limbus

Loupes magnifying lenses placed over glasses for fine work or optical surgery

Lumen cavity of a hollow organ or BV

Luminance amount of light emanating from an object and producing a sensation of brightness

Lymph (LIMpf) excess fluid & proteins left behind from the capillaries as they move from the arterial to the venous side

Lyse (LĪZ) rupture of a cell membrane and spilling of the intracellular contents

Lysozyme anti-bacterial enzyme found in normal tears - dissolves the coating of some bacteria

M

macro- large

Macrophage big eater - large mononuclear leukocyte involved in chronic If, mopping up cell debris present in granulomas

Macula an area of darker or changed pigmentation *wrt eyes* the yellow region in the centre of the retinal fundus surrounding the fovea *see Macula lutea*

Macula lutea an area of yellow pigmentation due to deposits of xanthophyll carotenoids yellow pigments - high in cholesterol in the retinal fundus **AKA Area Centralis** is a clinical term, and refers to the area observed when examining the retina, it is a yellow circle 6mm diameter of the retina bounded by the temporal retinal BV arcades & containing a thickened ganglion cell layer. It surrounds the fovea & foveola

Macular Degeneration a deterioration of the retina in the macular region of the retina there are 2 main types wet & dry - severely affects VA

Macular Hole small defect full thickness in the retina assoc. with VB retraction similar to a retinal tear but in the macular region

Macular Oedema AS Macular Edema swelling of the macular region of the retina - often due to If as in post cataract removal

Macular Pucker AKA Cellophane maculopathy puckering of the thin transparent preretinal layer which then interferes with VA

Maculopathy non-specific pathology of the macula

Madarosis (mad-ah-ROH-sis) AKA Ptilosis loss of eyelashes /eyebrows due to disease &/or excessive plucking – may be congenital

Major meridians refers to the meridians which have the highest & lowest optical power in astigmatism

-malacia softening

Malar (MAY-lar) cheek

Malignant uncontrolled usually pathological

Mandible from the verb to chew, hence, the movable lower jaw; ***adj.- mandibular.***

Manifest obvious apparent (≠ latent)

Manz glands conjunctival glands circling the cornea & producing mucin

Map-dot-fingerprint-dystrophy *see Epithelial basement membrane dystrophy*

Marcus Gun pupil a pupil which dilates very slowly when exposed to bright light - almost always accompanied by ↓ VA assoc. with ON disease – the normal pupil reacts to light rapidly, but is slower in reaction if the light is hone on the abnormal pupil *see also swinging flashlight test*

Marfan's syndrome *see Arachnodactyly*

Martegiani's area area over the surface of the ON head – where there is no vitreous adhesion – but surrounded by a ring of tight vitreous adhesion on its rim

Masquerade syndrome certain tumours in the eye will stimulate an apparent If disease of its adnexae

Maxilla the jaw-bone; now used only for the upper jaw; ***adj.- maxillary.***

Maxwell's spot perception of a bluish spot surrounded by a halo when a blue filter is placed before the eye – to test for macula function *see also Entopic Phenomenon*

Meatus a short passage; ***adj. meatal*** as in external acoustic meatus connecting the outer ear with the middle ear.

Medulla lowest part of the BStem connecting the Pons with the SC

Meibum (MĪ-bum) an oily secretion from the Meibomian glds (AKA tarsal glds) of the eye to lubricate the cornea

-megaly - enlargement

Meningioma tumour of the coverings of the brain – these extend along to the ON to the back of the EB and so may affect its integrity

Meningitis If of the meninges - the brain coverings

Meniscus *wrt eyes* crescent shaped body – tear-filld space b/n the CL & the cornea *(pl menisci)*

Mental relating to the chin (mentum = chin *not mens* = mind).

Meridian line around the EB through the ant. & post poles (AP, PP) at right angles to the Equator (E)

Mesial (MEEZ-ee-al) along the dental arch in the direction of the medial plane

Mesopic vision vision in low light involving rods *see also Dark adaptation (≠ Photopic vision)*

Mesodermal dysgenesis of the cornea *see Peter's anomaly*

Metamorphosia wavy distortion of vision

micro- small -

Micronystagmus small oscillations with eye fixation NAD unless larger *see Nystagmus*

Microphthalmos abnormally small eye with abnormal function *see also Nanophthalmos*

Microscopic pertaining to structures which are able to be viewed under the microscope

Midbrain upper part of the BStem contains the nuclei of CN III –VI with control function of papillary gazes

Midpupillary line AKA Pupillary axis line from the centre of the pupil to the visual focus pint

Migraine vascular blood disorder with cycle of vascular spasm & dilatation w/n the skull resulting in severe headache- nausea & visual &/or olfactory auras – maybe one-sided

> **Ocular/ ophthalmic** accompanied by lightning flashes and temporary VL
> **Ophthalmoplegic** accompanied by temporary ocular N palsies
> **Retinal** accompanied by severe VL ± headache

Miosis (MĪ-oh-sis) small pupils/ constricted pupils *adj miotic* used to describe medications which cause pupillary constriction *(≠ Mydriasis) see also Pupil*

© A. L. Neill

Molecule a neutral group of atoms held together by ionic or covalent bonds - however it is often also a term used for a charged polyatomic group which are technically *Radicals*

Moll glands sweat glands of the ELs

Molluscum contagiosum small wart-like lesion around the ELs caused by a virus and causing conjunctivitis

Monochromacy AKA Achromacy AKA Achromatism inability to distinguish colours

Monochromatic light of the one or narrow band frequency – one colour *see also Achromatic*

Monocular depth perception *see Parallax*

Monocular diplopia double vision from the one eye – sign of early cataracts or irregular corneas *see also Diplopia*

Monomers individual units of a larger structure - usually with the building up of extracellular fibres e.g. collagen *see also polymers*

Motor fusion corrective eye movements (vergences) that enable thee eyes to see a single image in a moving object – *see also Normal retinal correspondence*

Motor N AKA Efferent N N fibres which carry impulses away from the brain to cause a response – as in a muscle contraction eg CN III oculomotor N

Mucin (MEW-sin) secretion which acts as a protective lubricant from mucous glands

Mucosa (MEW-koh-zuh) tissue in the GIT immediately beneath the epithelial lining

Mucous AKA Mucoid *adj of mucus* as in mucous glands – glands which produce mucus

Mucus (MEW-kus) substance excreted by **Mucous** glands to lubricate food or protect mucosal surfaces *adj Mucoid / Mucous*

Müller cell AS Mueller cell (MEW-ler) supportive retinal cell spans the length of the retina and supplies nutrient to the specialized sensory cells of vision

Müller's muscle samooth muscle sheets which provide tone for the ELs & circular muscle fibres of the innermost part of **Ciliaris**

Munson's sign bowing of the lower EL when looking down due to keratoconus

Mural cells cells of the retinal capillary walls

Muscae Volitantes (MUS-kee vol-inTAN-tuz) black or dark specs seen when looking at a very bright area such as the sky, caused by remnants of the hyaloids a & its branches in the VB *see also Floaters*

Muscle of Riolan AKA Pars Ciliaris part of the orbicularis ocular m – which inserts in the medial canthus and allows complete closure on the nasal side of the eye

Muscle cone *wrt eye* – the post. cone of the orbit surrounded by the EOM, containing the BVs & Ns.

Muscle sheath AKA Intermusclular membrane CT covering of all the muscles which allow for free movement over each other

Mydriasis large pupil / dilated pupil *adj mydriatic* used to describe the medications which cause the dilatation of the pupil (↗ *Miosis*)

Myelin (MĬ-e-lin) fatty sheath covering N fibres to ↑ nerve impulse speed & intensity *adj myelinated*

Myokymia (MĬ-oh-KĬ-me-uh) spasmodic twitching of an EL m assoc. with fatigue

Myopia (MY-oh-pee-uh) **AKA Nearsightedness** inability to see objects far away a form of "over focusing" , due to the focal point falling in front of the retinal surface, ie the EB is too long

The corneal : retinal length ratio is incorrect, due to :

Overcurvature of the cornea – *refractive myopia*

Overcurvature of the lens - *index myopia*

Overcontraction of the ciliary m – seen in school children studying close work for too long – *School myopia*

Expansion of the EB length – with age, weakening of the sclera ↑ IOP – **progressive myopic degeneration**

Myositis If of the muscles

Myotomy resection – removal of a muscle

N

Naevus AS Nevus small mole, benign skin Tm, may also occur in the ocular Ts in the RPE

Naevus of Ota AKA Oculodermal melanocytosis pigmented area on the cheek ELs forehead or nose

Nanophthalmos abnormally small eye with normal function *see* **Microphthalmos**

Naris nostrils *pl. Nares*

Narrow angle AKA Shallow angle shallower than normal angle b/n the iris & the corner – important bc this interferes with the draining of the ant. chamber → ↑ IOP → VL i.e. Glaucoma

Nasal sinuses a term for the collective spaces from: the Ethmoid, Frontal, Maxillary & Sphenoid bones most of which flank the orbit

Near point the point at which the eye is fully focused to the maximum of its accommodation

Near reflex collective term for the reflexes need to occur when focusing on an approaching object: accommodation, convergence & miosis (pupil constriction)

Near-sightedness *see Myopia*

Necrosis cell or T death

Necrotizing scleritis severe If of the sclera assoc. with other degenerative inflammatory diseases eg RA

neo - (NEE-oh) new

Neoplasm new abnormal growth for no apparent reason – usually malignant

Neovascularization formation of new abnormal BVs usually in or under the retina or iris generally as a response to perceived or actual anoxia which may be induced by retinal BV degeneration as in DM, blockage of the retinal vessels, MD etc.

Nerve fibre bundle defect arc-shaped blindspot (scotoma) caused by damage to the retinal N fibre layers

Nerve fibre bundle layer of the retina (NFL) innermost retinal layer i.e. next to the VB, containing the axons of all the Ns towards the ON head at the OD in a characteristic pattern

Neuritis If of a N

> **Optic** If of the ON ss rapid VL pain on movement of the EB and central VFD

> **Retrobulbar** If of the ON behind the OD ss → VA assoc. in both cases with demyelinating disease e.g. multiple sclerosis

Neuroblastoma malig. Tm of the SymNS in infants spread to the eye from the adrenal medulla presenting as swollen bleeding ELs & eyes with proptosis

Neurofibromatosis AKA von Reckinghausen's disease a phakomatosis (disease with small Tms of the skin & CNS) with bony defects in the orbital bones

Neuromuscular junction the junction b/n motor N fibre & muscle cell

Neuro-ophthalmology science of the eye & brain interrelationships

Neuropathy non-IF diseases of the NS

Neuroretinitis If of the retina near or assoc. with the ON

Neuroretinopathology AKA Neuroretinopathy non-If retinal pathology occurring near the ON

Neurotomy cutting of a N or group of Ns

Neurotransmitter chemical substance generated by N cells to communicate intercellularly – ie to transmit the N impulse from one cell to another, which maybe b/n N cells or N cells & muscle cells eg acetylcholine, adrenalin (AKA epinephrine) & nor-adrenalin

Neutral density filter a filter placed before the eyes to ↓ the incident light – used to differentiate amblyopia – if reversible the filter will improve or have no effect on VA – but if there is functional deficit the filter will just ↓ VA eg sunglasses will not help or improve vision in an affected eye

Neutrophil AKA Polymorphonuclear leucocyte (PMN) WBC with multi-lobed nucleus major cell response in acute If episodes the neutrophil leaves the BS & becomes a PMN

Nevus AS Naevus

Nictitiation winking or blinking – derived for the membrane in some animals where they have a 3rd EL which sweeps laterally across the eye

Nidus site of origin of grth development or cancer spread *(pl nidi)*

Night blindness AKA Nyctalopia inefficient dark adaptation which results in severe ↓ VA in dim light

Night Vision AKA Rod vision AKA Scotopic vision the amount of VA in dim light maximal adaptation occurs after 30 mins *see also Dark Adaptation*

Nodal point AKA Optical centre ref point on the principal axis - line along which the incident light is not refracted

Non-Comitant Strabismus eye deviation differs with different gazes *see also Strabismus*

Non-optic reflex eye movements eye movements initiated by the inner ear or head movements

Normal retinal correspondence binocular adaptation of the retinas so that a single binocular image is seen from the fovea of each eye *see also harmonious abnormal retinal correspondence, unharmonious retinal correspondence*

Notch an indentation in the margin of a structure.

Nucha the nape or back of the neck *adj.- nuchal.*

Nucleolus (NEW-klee-oh-lus) little nucleus - a small unbound collection of RNA w/in the nucleus which varies in size, shape and presence due to the activity of the cell. It is the site of rRNA synthesis and dispersement, & the assembly of ribosomes. It appears as a darkly staining spot(s) in the nucleus *pl nucleoli*

Nyctalopia *see Night blindness*

Nystagmus involuntary eye movement of the EB in any direction, with one motion faster than the other "returning movement"

O

Objective lens - in an optical instrument the objective is the furthest lens from the ocular lens

Obtunded made dull, ↓ sensitivity

Occiput the prominent convexity of the back of the head Occiputum = Occipital bone - this is the bone opposite the occipital lobes of the brain - the site of visual perception adj. occipital

Occludable referring to the angle of the ant. chamber & the iris which may be blocked by the anterior iris and so stop the flow of the aqueous fluid and lead to glaucoma

Occluded pupil AKA Occlusio Pupillo covering of the pupillary opening with a membrane after an inflammatory disease and which blocks the flow of the AH from the post. chamber to the ant. chamber

Occlusion opposition of the teeth when closed = bite

Occult hidden

oculo-/ocular pertaining to the eye

Ocular Adnexae structures surrounding the eye e.g. EL, eyebrow, eyelash *see also Adnexa*

Ocular Albinism defect in the pigment of the iris & choroid assoc. with ↓ VA, photophobia &nystagmus

Ocular biometry measurements of the eye eg the axial length

Ocular Bobbing disordered spontaneous fast downwards jerking of both eyes with slow return - assoc. with BStem disease

Ocular Dysmetria (dis-MEE-tree-uh) AKA Ocular flutter AKA Ocular bobbing uncoordinated eye movement with overshooting of the eyes when focusing until a stable point is reached assoc. with cerebellar disease

Ocular media cornea, aqueous fluids, lens & VB - the transparent media of the eye

Ocular myoclonus rapid side to side eye movements , assoc. with the pons or pretectal BStem diseases

Ocular Pemphigus (PEM-fig-us) progressive blistering & scarring of the mm (conjunctiva) of the eye, causes extreme drying & scarring of the sclera & cornea

Ocular Torticollis abnormal head tilt to compensate for EOM changes

Oculo-cardiac reflex ↓ HR following manipulation of the EB

Oculo-cephalic reflex AKA Vestibulo-ocular reflex involuntary eye rotation in the opposite direction from the head rotation to maintain fixation on an object which maybe abnormal as in Doll's eyes

Oculo-digital reflex constant rubbing or pushing of the eyes by blind children

Oculo-respiratory reflex cessation of breathing as the EOM are tugged in eye surgery

Oculodermal melanocytosis AKA Ota's naevus AKA Naevus of Ota pigmented lesions on: the cheek, ELs, forehead or nose

Oculodynia AKA Oculomalagia pain in & around the eyes

Oculogyric crisis involuntary spasmodic upward movement of the eyes assoc with basal ganglia disease

Oculomotor apraxia inability to move the eyes voluntary eye movements - resulting in head thrusting to find the correct gaze

Oculomotor decussation the crossing over to the other side of the fibres controlling the horizontal gaze from CN III / IV at the level b/n 3rd & 4th cranial nuclei - hence lesions below this cause horizontal gaze deficits on the same side but above this on the contralateral side

Oedema (eh-DEEM-uh) AS Edema swelling due to fluid

Oedipism (EE-dip-ism) AKA Self-enucleation a severe form of self harm where the person removes their own eye(s) after Oedipus after realizing that he had unwittingly slept with his mother gouges his eyes out with her golden brooches

Oligodendrocyte supportive glial cell in the ON and CNS produces myelin to protect N processes *see also Astrocyte*

One & one half syndrome BStem lesion of the medial longitudinal fasciculus & paramedian pontine reticular formation, resulting in the inability to gaze in one direction horizontally *see also Oculomotor Decussation*

Opacity quality of being opaque *see also Translucent* ≠ *Transparent*

Opaque solid not transparent, material which blocks the transmission of light

Open globe injury full thickness injury to the cornea &/or sclera

-opathy pertaining to disease

-opia pertaining to the eyes / eyesight

Operculum cover / lid *wrt eye* flap of torn retina - free or attached

Ophritis AS Ophyritis dermatitis of the skin around the eyebrow

Optic Chiasm *see Chiasm* point at which the ON of each eye form a cross and appear to "cross over" – note the relationship to the hypothalamus & the pituitary gld

Ophthalmology (OPF-thal-mol-oh-gee) study of the eye & its associated structures

Ophthalmoplegia general term for the restriction or inability to move the eyes through full ROM

> **external** - acquired paralysis of the EOM
> **internal** - loss of function w/n the eye
> **painful** - If condition with restricted movement of the EB **AKA Tolosa-Hunt syndrome**
> **total** - combination of the above

Ophthalmoscope an instrument used to view inside the EB. The commonest is that illustrated below which uses a direct light source. The examiner focuses on the retina, ON, macula and other internal structures using different lenses. The best results can be obtained after first dilating the pupil using mydriatic drops.

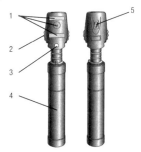

1 – site for examiner – aperture & head rests, 2 – focus wheel brings lenses into view to allow for focusing on the retina 3 – indicates the lens strength 4- handle & 5 – light source.

Opsin colourless protein (+vitamin A) found in the outer segments of the rod & cone cells used to change the light energy into electrical energy to form the N impulse

Opsoclonus sequence of jerky horizontal movements in both eyes assoc with cerebellar disease *see also Ocular flutter, Dysmetria*

Optic atrophy ON degeneration manifesting as pallor of the OD

Optic disc (OD) AKA Optic Nerve Head AKA Optic Papilla the visual portion of the ON - 1.5mm in diameter - note the term *optic papilla* is no longer used

Optic nerve (ON) the 2nd cranial N - this is the special sensory N which carries the impulses from the retina to the brain

Optic Nerve Pit AKA Optic Nerve Colomba incomplete fusion of the foetal fissure in development

Optic Neuritis AKA Papillitis AKA Retrobulbar neuritis If of the ON ss VL, pain on movement

Optic radiation AKA Geniculo-calcarine tract tract in the VP b/n lateral geniculate body & the calcarine fissure

Optical axis AKA Principal axis line through the optical centres of any lens

Optineurin protein found in the ON & CNS - plays a protective role in the health of the Nc

Optotype the letters, number or pictures printed on the charts used for VA testing - the commonest of these is the Snellen chart. Others include: **the E chart** - with rolling Es whose orientation has to be identified or **the Allen chart** where images are used

Ora Serrata anterior edge of the retina 6.5mm behind the limbus with a tooth-like edge, non-visual

Orbit AKA Socket a circle; the name given to the bony socket in which the eyeball rotates, *adj - orbital.*

Orbital Apex narrow innermost part of the pyramid shaped bony orbit

Orbital cellulitis If of the orbit often due to spread from Ins in the adjacent sinuses

Orbital fat pads the 4 fat pads lying b/n the 4 Recti m

Orbital periosteum AKA Periorbita adherent outer CT layer of the bony orbit

Orbital septum AKA Palpebral fascia CT which supports the EL & periorbital fascia, separating the orbital contents from the EL contents

Organ a group of tissues & cells which are bound together to perform a specific function

Orifice (or-EE-fiss) an opening.

ortho- straight

Orthofusor booklet of stereoscopic images used to try & improve binocular vision in deviated eyes

Orthophoria straight eyes w/o any deviation *adj orthophoric (≠ Strabismus)*

Orthopnea (or-THOP-nee-uh) difficulty in breathing when lying down

Orthoptics the study & Tx of the defects of binocular visual function or of the ocular muscles

Orthotropic absence of eye deviation but w/o image fusion

Ota's Naevus *see Oculodermal melanocytosis*

Otolith apparatus inner ear mechanism by which the eyes remain in the same position despite head movement

-otomy pertaining to cutting or opening a tissue

Outer Retina AKA Retinal pigmented epithelium (RPE) inner choroid layer which nourishes the visual cells of the retina

Overwear syndrome corneal changes from overuse of CLs epithelial erosion resulting in corneal swelling

P

Pachometry AKA Pachymetry measurement of the corneal thickness + ant. chambre depth

Palate a roof *adj.- palatal or palatine.*

Palinopsia AKA Visual Preservation persistence of an image after looking away

Palpebra pertaining to the EL *adj palpebral*

Palpebral commissure *see Canthus*

Palpebral fascia AKA Orbital septum prevents the orbital contents from protruding

Palpebral fissure the "slit" opening b/n the upper and lower ELs

Pannus infiltration of BVs into the cornea

Panophthalmitis If of the entire EB and its contents

Papilla (e) (PAP-ill-uh (ee)) outpouching – point generally with an opening as in the duodenal papilla wrt eyes generally referring to enlarged conjunctival follicles distinguished by their own core BVs (1) & CT fibrous septa (2) in the collections of lymphoid T (3) + other long standing If cells e.g. macrophages (4) of severe allergic conjunctivitis or chronic longstanding conjunctivitis of CL overuse appearing under the palpebral conjunctival epithelium (5) *see also Follicle*

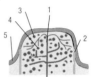

Papillitis If of the head of the ON

Papilloedema is bilateral OD elevation due to ↑intracranial P. It is not a true oedema or swelling but rather a damning of the axoplasmic flow because of ↑perineural P.

Parallax phenomenon of seeing the object from different perspectives and thus being able determine distance & depth *binocular* - use of 2 sources cf 2 eyes; *motion* - use of different speed perception slower from distant objects and faster with closer objects *see also Depth perception*

Parenchyma (PA-ren-KY-muh) main component of an organ when it is highly cellular e.g. the liver

Paresis weakness / partial paralysis

Parietal (pa-RYE-et-al) pertaining to the outer wall of a cavity from paries, a wall.

Parotid (pa-ROT-id) pertaining to a region beside or near the ear

pars a part of

Perimeter *in the eye* the edge of the VF

Perimetry measurement of the full extent of the VF

Periosteum layer of fascial tissue, CT on the outside of compact bone not present on articular (joint) surfaces *see endostium*

Periorbita *see Orbital periosteum*

Peripheral vision ability to perceive the presence & movement of objects outside the direct line of vision

Pctrous pertaining to a rock / rocky / stony *adj. Petrosal*

phago (FAY-goh) to eat

phako AS phaco- (FAY-koh) pertaining to the lens (in the eye)

Phagocytosis the active ingestion of larger particles & their digestion

Phakoemulsification surgical procedure using ultrasonic vibration to break up a cataract into small fragments & emulsify them in order to suck these fragments out of the lens capsule while preserving the capsule as much as possible - replacing extracapsular extraction

Phi phenomenon apparent movement of an object b/n rapid succession of image exposures as in movies - or in misaligned eyes covered and regarding the same object

-phimosis (fim-OH-sis) *wrt the eye* a constricted opening of the ELs

Phoria (FOR-ee-uh) *see Hetrerophoria*

-phoria *wrt the eye* a tendency to ....*see also -tropia which is a manifest or evident change in the eye for example in squints*

Phosphene seeing stars, light perceived w/o any light, maybe triggered by optic neuritis or irritation of the retina, other parts of the OP or very loud sounds

Phosphorylation addition of 1 or more phosphate radicals to a structure - usually protein

Photophobia abnormal sensitivity to light

photo- (FOh-toh) pertaining to light

Photocoagulation laser procedure on intraocular structures to burn or ablate them - ie new BVs on the retina

Photometry measurement of light

Photopic vision daylight vision involving mainly the cones (*≠ Mesopic vision*)

Photopsia appearance of sparks or flashes w/n the eye due to retinal irritation – not from a light source

Phlyctenule (flik-TEN-yool) a wedge-shaped lymphoid T deposit at the edge of the cornea in reaction to bacterial conjunctivitis

Phthsis bulbi (TI-sis BULB-ï) end stage EB after protracted disease of the EB, characterized by small EB as the CB stops producing aqueous humour

pilo- (PĬ-loh) hair

Pigment clumping & Pigment drop-out site of irregular pigmentation in the retina due to vitreous tugs, past retinal tears or past vitreous adherent areas - dropout is more severe than clumping - usually reversible after weeks to months

Pilomatrixoma hairy mole on the face

Pinhole test testing the VA while eliminating the factors of RE & intraocular opacities *see also Dilated Pinhole test*

Pinguecula(e) (pin-GWEK-yu-luh) *(Lt. fat, grease)* a yellow / white deposit(s) found near the limbus due to collagen degradation & elastin proliferation in response to ↑ UV exposure DD Pterygium common in > 40yos

Pink eye AKA Conjunctivitis *see also Red eye*

Pisciform (PI-sih-form) fish-shaped

Plaque (PLARK) small differentiated area on the body or BV wall eg fatty &/or calcium deposits on an artery wall - atheroma *wrt eye* - plaques seen on the arterioles of the retinal arterioles may indicate BV disease of the retina

Plasma is blood w/o its cellular components *see also Serum*

pleo- (PLEE-oh) AKA poly- (POL-ee) many generally referring to shapes

Plexus network of either Ns or BVs

Plica (e) (PLEE-ku/kay) fold (s) generally fixed folds with a CT stem to fix their shape

Plica Lacrimalis *see Hasner's valve*

Plica Semilunaris a semicircular fold of the bulbar conjunctiva (1) at the media canthus to permit extended lateral movement of the EB and facilitate drainage via the LA - remnant of the nictitating membrane (3rd EL) *see also Canthus, Caruncle*

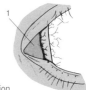

Polarization light which is in only one plane of vibration

Poliosis depigmentation of the eyelashes assoc. with sympathetic ophthalmia

poly- many

Polycoria more than one pupillary opening in the iris

Polymegathism increased size of corneal endothelial cells

Polymers repeated "monomer" units as in several monomers of the collagen fibre placed together but not enough to be a complete fibre *see also Monomer*

Polyopia many images seen in early cataract or severe astigmatism

Pontine lesions tumour in the pons area of the BStem which may affect adjacent areas assoc. CN VI palsies, lack of corneal reflex & sensation - CN V_1 involvement, difficulty in vorcions & nystagmus

Posterior chambre space filled with AH anterior to the lens and posterior to the iris

Power measure of the RP of a lens

Preretinal area b/n the anterior of the retina & the face of the VB, area ↑ with age

pres- (PREZ-) associated with age

Presbyopia (PREZ-by-oh-pee-uh) "old sight" shortsightedness associated with age - inability to focus on close items

Pretectal area junctional zone at the top of the midbrain which contains the centres for pupillary reactions, vergence movements & upward gaze

Primary position the normal position of the EBs in their sockets - note the lateral orbital walls are if extended at right angles to each other

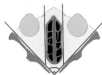

Primary visual cortex AKA Occipital lobe

Prince rule instrument to measure the point at which objects go out of focus as the object approaches

Prism wedge-shaped transparent medium which bends light rays towards it base

Prism Diopters a measure of the mal-alignment b/n the 2 eyes not equal to or the same as Diopters, which are a measure of RF
1 prism diopter brings the light focused at 1m - 1cm closer

Process a general term describing any marked projection or prominence as in the mandibular process.

Prolapse slipping of an object out of its normal position *wrt eyes* lens prolapse

Proliferative retinopathy retinal deterioration in which there is neovascularization of the retinal BVs often seen in DM leading to →Hg, → retinal traction, →retinal detachment & VL

Proliferative vitreoretinopathy AKA Massive preretinal proliferation retinopathy involving the VB & so further distorting VA ***see also Macular Pucker***

Proptosis AKA Eye dislocation AKA Eye luxation AKA Eye protrusion is a condition resulting in forward displacement and entrapment of the eye from behind by the ELs. The condition is also known as **eye dislocation & eye luxation**. It is a common result of head trauma & P exerted on the front of the neck or Tms behind or w/n the EB.

Protanopia inability to see red

Proximal closer to the axial skeleton (**≠ Distal**)

Pseudophakic (SEW-doh-fay-kik) implanted prosthetic lens in the eye (generally due to cataracts)

Pterygium (TER-rij-ee um) AKA Surfer's eye *(Lt wing or wedge-shaped* condition where there is a triangular overgrowth of the nasal conjunctiva which may be cosmetically distressing but is not important unless the growth continues onto the cornea and affects the vision

Ptilosis *see Madarosis*

Ptosis (TOH-sis) *(Gk a fall)* drooping of an organ or structure e.g. the upper &/or lower ELs *(adj ptotic)*

> **aponeurotic** due to a slippage of the LPS from the EL membrane - commonest form seen in the elderly
> **congenital dystrophic** generally hereditary
> **mechanical** drooping 2° to a Tm or other interfering phenomenon
> **myogenic** due to malfunction of the LPS often assoc with systemic disease
> **neurogenic** 2° to CN III palsy
> **traumatic**
> **upside down** lower EL sitting too high, 2° t° sympathetic malfunction seen in Horner's syndrome
> *see also Bell's palsy, Blepharoptosis*

Pulfrich phenomenon delay in the transmission of the visual impulses from 1 eye than the other & assoc with diplopia - lower the illumination in the faster eye to normalize

Punctum (a) external orifices of the upper & lower canaliculi of the LA - surrounded by a papilla

Pupil the opening of the EB beneath the cornea to allow light via the lens to pass into the retina. There are a number of variations functional & pathological - 1 dilated / mydriatic, 2 constricted / miotic pupils; 3 full / sector, 4 peripheral iridectomies , 5 congenital colomba; iridodialysis & 6 synchiae / iridal adhesions

 1
 2
 3
 4
5
 6
 6

Pupillary distance (PD) AKA Interpupillary distance the distance b/n the centre of the 2 pupils

Pupillotonia *see Adie's pupil*

Purkinje images the 4 images seen when shining the light onto closed ELs to see one's own retinal BVs

Purkinje shift shift from the light to dark vision & so sensitivity moves from 555 nm to 507 nm as the rods take over the main sensory visual perception

Purulent (PEW-roo-lent) containing puss

Pyogenic (PĬ-oh-jen-ik) producing pus

Q

Quadrantanopia AKA
Quadrantanopsia VFD involving a
quadrant or quarter of the VF in each eye

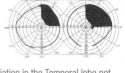

> **inferior assoc.** with Parietal lobe
> involvement
>
> **superior** AKA pie in the sky
>
> assoc. with inf. fibres of the optic radiation in the Temporal lobe not
> necessarily the same if due to a lesion there may be asymmetry as
> demonstrated here

Quadrantic defect VFD in 1/4 of the VF

R

Radicals charged atomic particles or charged polyatomic groups which may
be bound to larger molecules or freely disassociated and "unbound" - **_free
radicals_** - refer to an unbound charged ions or molecules - and are highly
reactive

Raphe (RAF-ay) line of joint b/n 2 halves, generally of bone or muscles for
example a fibrous raphe in the tongue allowing for muscle insertion

**Rapid Eye movements (REM) AKA Saccades AKA Fast eye
movements** fast eye movements of about 60s seen in the dream state of
sleeping

Recess a secluded area or pocket; a small cavity set apart from a main cavity.

Rectus straight, erect

Red Eye term used to describe any condition where the eye has dilated BVs
& appears "red" - most inflammatory conditions **_see also Conjunctivitis,
Pink eye_**

Red Reflex the normal red glow emerging from the pupil when the interior is
illuminated - any difference indicates pathology

Refixation fast involuntary eye movements as the eye shifts from one object
to another - or tries to follow a very fast object

Reflex involuntary reaction to a stimulus _wrt eyes_
types - **blink, corneal, oculo-cardiac, oculo-digital, pupillary ,
vestibulo-ocular**

Reflex tearing crying in response to ocular stimulation eg touching the
cornea

Refraction bending of light via a lens
> **cycloplegic** refraction in the eye w/o the influence of the lens
> **manifest** refraction with the influence of the lens

Refractive error (RE) AKA Ametropia an optical defect that prevents light rays from being brought to a single focus

Reiter's syndrome syndrome of uveitis / iritis, arthritis & urethritis

Restrictive syndromes eye deviation caused by mechanical obstruction of the EOM &/or their fibrous sheaths

Retina innermost coat of the eye, consisting of the sensory retina which interacts with the RPE *adj retinal*

Retinal Correspondence the melding of the 2 images from each eye into one image

Retinal detachment a separation of the sensory retina from it BS an supportive epithelial cells

Retinitis If of the retina

Retinitis pigmentosa a hereditary degeneration of the retina

Retinitis proliferans If of the retina assoc. with neovascularization & fibrosis

Retinoblastoma Tm of the retina, which will track back through the ON if untreated - commonest childhood ocular malignancy

Retinochoroiditis If of the retina + choroid assoc with toxoplasmosis

Retinol AKA Vitamin A stored in the liver and used by the rods & cones in the synthesis of their photosensitive pigment

Retinopathy non-specific disease and degeneration of the retina
types: **cellophane** *see Macular puckering*
    central serous smooth blister-like in the macula which results in retinal detachment
    chloroquin drug induced retinopathy, forming rings around the macula -with VL which is reversible in the early stages
    circinate (sir-sin-ayt) ring formation of exudates around the macula
    diabetic non-proliferative -moving to proliferative neovascularization & fibrosis
    familial exudative vitreal weeping exudate from the retina causing neovascularization similar to **premature retinopathy**
    flavimacular AKA Stargardt's disease characterized by yellow flecks in the retina
    haemorrhagic massive intraretinal Hgs with dilated & engorged veins with papilloedema due to blockage of the retinal BVs
    hypertensive related to hypertension *see copper & silver wiring*
    neuro- involvement of the ON w/o BV involvement
    Purtscher's cottonwool retinal patched assoc with sudden transient ↑BP reversible
    sickle-cell neovascularization and retinal BV blockage changes
    solar damage from looking at the sun / or other bright light
    tapeto- hereditary grp of retinal degenerative diseases

Retinoschisis (ret-in-oh-SKEE-sis) splitting of the retina resulting in partial or complete "hole" formation in the peripheral retina- does not result in central VL present in ~3% of the population

Retrolental behind the lens

Rhexis (REK-sis) breaking of an organ or BV

Rhinus/rhino- (RYE-noh) pertaining to the nose

Rhodospin AKA Visual Purple visual pigment of the rod cells, dependent upon vitamin A, and responsible for most of the low illumination vision of the eye

Riddoch phenomenon ability to perceive a moving object but not a still one

Ridge elevated bony growth often roughened.

Right gaze verticals term used to describe eye up & down when looking to the R - (RIR, RSR, LIO & LSO)

Rosacea (ROZ-ay-SHEE-uh) skin disease of the face cheeks & ELs which may involve the eye, drying the cornea eg **Rosacea keratitis** & inflaming other uveal components

Rose Bengal purplish dye routinely used to detect corneal defects

Rostral towards the anterior/front (of the brain)

Roth Spots *see Spots*

Rotundum round

Rubeosis Iridis (ROOB-ee-oh-sis IR-id-is) formation of new BVs & fibrosis on the ant. surface of the iris in late stage of retinopathy from other causes

Ruga (e) (ROO-gu/ gay) folds – generally more mobile and less structured than Plicae – can be flattened as in Stomach

S

Sac soft-walled cavity

Saccades AKA Rapid Eye Movements (REM) voluntary quick eye movements in the same direction - mechanism for fixation, refixation & the fast phase of optokinetic nystagmus initiated by the frontal lobes of the brain (Brodmann area 8) *see also Slow Eye Movements*

Sagittal an arrow, the sagittal suture is notched posteriorly, making it look like an arrow by the lambdoid sutures. *wrt eye* sagittal plane is from ant. to post. pole

Salus sign retinal vein deflection at a crossing of an artery & vein so that it crosses more perpendicularly one of the signs of ↑IOP possibly 2° to hypertension

Salzmann's degeneration non-If degeneration of the cornea ss pearl grey nodules on the edge of the cornea

Sattler's veil *see Corneal bedewing*

Scaphoid (SKAY-foyd) boat-shaped *wrt eyes* preretinal Hg with a flattened top

Scheerer's phenomenon *see Blue squiggles*

Scheiner principle when viewing a distant light source through 2 pinholes - the normal eye will see only one spot but the eye with a RE will see 2 spots - ie the unfocused eye will see a double image

Schwalbe's line peripheral edge of Descemet's membrane in the cornea

Schwann cell cell of the PNS responsible for myelination similar to the glial cells of the CNS

Scissors motion bserved crossing light beams in eye examination indicating RE of the EB

Scintillating scotoma flashes of light in rings assoc with occiptial lobe disorders & migraine

Sclera AKA Tunica Fibrosa Oculi the white of the EB - a thick CT layer continuous with the cornea & site of EOM insertion

Scleral spur mass of scleral fibres bordered in ant. by the canal of Schlemm & post. by the Ciliaris

Scleral Trabeculae AKA Trabecular meshwork CT fibres mesh at the irideoscleral junction to allow for the drainage of the ant. chamber

Sclerosis hardening *adj sclerotic*

Scleritis deep If of the sclera accompanied by episcleritis (surface If of the sclera), severe pain, weakening & swelling of the sclera may result in VL
types: **anterior** - in front of the equator
    brawny - widespread swollen gelatinous
    nodular - localized tender lumps
    posterior - behind the equator
    see also episcleritis

Scotoma a defect in the VF
types: **angio-** defect due to shadow of a BV
    annular - ring form
    arcuate AKA Bjerrum AKA simitar - arch caused by N fibre damage as in glaucoma
    central - in the region of the macula >5% will cause profound VA loss
    centrocaecal - central + additional region - assoc with toxic damage to the ON
    junction - central + temporal scotomas in each eye due to P on the chiasm
    negative - found on examination - patient unaware ≠ **positive**
    paracentral - not in the macula region
    physiologic AKA of Mariotte - ↑ normal blindspot >7° because of lack of photoreceptor cells near ON
    relative - incomplete VFD
    scintillating - flashing rings of lights assoc with migraines *pl scotomata*

Scotopic adaptation AKA Dark adaptation adaptation to low levels of light which is perceived only by rods

Secluded pupil AKA Seclusio Pupillae blockage of the post. chamber drainage

Second grade fusion phenomenal fusion of 2 images b/n normal & deviated eyes to allow perception of a single image, by moving the main focus off the fovea in the deviated eye

Second sight phenomenon of ability to read in previous presbyopia due to crystalline lens central focusing

Sella Turcica bony pocket in the base of the skull b/n & behind the orbits

Semilunar fold AKA Plica Semilunaris crescent-shaped fleshy mound of conjunctiva in the nasal canthus

Senescence (SEN-ess-ens) signs associated with aging e.g. in a cell the accumulation of lipofuscin is related to age

Separation difficulty AKA Crowding phenomenon difficulty in reading a line of letters but can read a single letter due to functional amblyopia

Septum a division

Serum (blood) is blood plasma w/o the clotting factors i.e. it is acellular fluid with fewer proteins & cannot clot

Silver wiring advanced form of copper wiring thickening of the retinal arterioles with ↑ BP & atherosclerosis

Sicca (SEE-ka) AKA Dry Eye syndrome AKA Keratitis AKA Sjogren's syndrome cluster of ss assoc with lack of tear film -itchiness, FB feeling grittiness, assoc with women > 50yo

Siderosis ss assoc with retained iron FB in the eye - a brown ring around the cornea, brown opacity developing in the cornea etc.

Sinus (SĬN-us) a space usually w/in a bone lined with mm, such as the frontal & maxillary sinuses in the head, (also, a modified BV usually vein with an enlarged lumen for blood storage & containing no or little muscle in its wall). Sinuses may contain air, blood, lymph, pus or serous fluid depending upon location & health of the subject *adj.- sinusoid.*

Sinus Venosus Sclerae AKA Schlemm's canal *see Canal of Schlemm*

Skull the skull refers to all of the bones that comprise the head.

Slit lamp biomicroscope AKA Slit lamp table top microscope allowing cornea, iris &lens to be seen layer by layer with a rectangular light beam in the LP *see also Confocal Microscope*

Slow eye movements smooth simultaneous movements of both eyes in the same or opposite directions <50°/s see Brodman area 19 (≠ REM), saccades

Snellen chart a chart used to determine central VA - consisting of numbers &/or letters of designated sizes *see also Allen cards*

Snowballs sign coarse cellular clumps w/n the VB assoc with post. uveitis & sarcoid

Soft exudates *see Cotton wool spots*

Solar maculopathy AKA Eclipse blindness central scotoma with VL from looking at the sun

Spheroid degeneration chronic If of the cornea due to exposure to UV light, white spots of collagen degeneration fibres on the cornea

Sphincter ring of muscle around a tube or opening, generally but not always, composed of skeletal muscle

Spine a thorn **adj. - spinous** descriptive of a sharp, slender process/ protrusion commonly used regarding the spinous processes of the VBs

Spiral of Tillaux AKA Contact Spiral imaginary line connecting all the EOM insertions on the sclera - showing the fact that the Recti are inserted further & further from the limbus from the MR (MR,IR, LR & SR) around to balance their actions ranging b/n 5-8mm - note the variation in the tendon lengths as well.

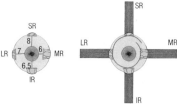

Splanchnocranium refers to the facial bones of the skull.

"Spots" in ophthalmology

> **Bitot's spot** - white, foamy area of keratinising squamous metaplasia of bulbar conjunctiva, assoc. with Vitamin A deficiency.
> **Brushfield spot** - whitish grey spot in peripheral iris, seen in Down's syndrome.
> **Elschnig spot** - yellow patches overlying area of choroidal infarction in ↑BP
> **Fischer-Khunt spot** - senile scleral plaque(s), area of hyalinised sclera ant. to the insertion of the rectus m
> **Fuch's spot** - RPE hyperplasia - dark lesions near the macula in pathological myopia.
> **Gunn's dot** - light reflections from ILM around the OD & macula
> **Horner-Trantras Dot** - collections of eosinophils at limbus in allergic conjunctivitis.
> **Kayes' dot** - subepithelial infiltrates seen in corneal graft rejection
> **Mittendorf's dot** - whitish spot at post. lens surface, remnant of hyaloid a
> **Roth spots** - Hgs with white centres, seen in severe anaemia, collagen vascular disorders.

-stoma to do with the mouth

Squamous cell carcinoma (SCC) skin cancer derived from squamous epithelial cells - may occur wherever there is an epithelial layer and take many forms.

Squint *see Strabismus*

Starburst perception of a point light as a star partic at night due to intraocular opacities - usually cataracts

Strabismus AKA Cross-eyed AKA Deviation AKA Squint AKA Heterotropia AKA Tropia (≠ orthophoric) condition of mal-alignment of the eyes generally due to the EOM - manifest deviation *see also Amblyopia*

Staphyloma a thinned part of the coat of the eye causing protrusion

***Stroma* (STROH-mu)** underlying T background may have various structures but is often equivalent to lamina propria (LP) *wrt eye* - **corneal** the fibrous middle layer comprising >90% of the corneal T, **iridal** the pigmented cells which coat & make up the bulk of the iris

Stye *see Hordeolum*

Subconjunctival haemorrhage *see Hyposphagma*
B from the conjunctival BVs accumulating in the conjunctiva, which stops abruptly at the limbus & does not involve the cornea, but may extend into the ELs

Subcutaneous under the skin, but has come to mean dermal - i.e. subepithelial

Subjunctive movement *see Gaze movement*

Submucosa deep to the mucosa

Surfer's eye *see Pterygium*

Sulcus (i) (SUL-kus/kee) long wide groove often due to a BV indentation, furrow cf in the brain wrt eye **-ciliary** to drain the blood from the EB, **grey** the groove separating the conjunctiva and EL skin

Superior above

Superior palpebral fissure upper EL fold

Suture the saw-like edge of a cranial bone that serves as joint b/n bones of the skull.

Swinging Flashlight test *see Marcus Gunn pupil*

Sylvian aqueduct syndrome *see Dorsal midbrain syndrome*

syn- together i.e. the close proximity of or fusion of 2 structures

Symbelpharon (sim-BLEF-ar-on) abnormal adhesion b/n the palpebral & bulbar conjunctiva

Sympathetic Ophthalmia AKA Sympathetic uveitis granulomatous If of the uvea as a late sequelea of penetrating eye ly - note rarely a similar uveitis will occur in the other unaffected eye months later *see also Dalen-Fuch's nodules, Poliosis*

Synchysis scintillans (sin-KEE-sis SIN-til-anz) AKA Cholesterolosis Bulbi formation of asymptomatic white cholesterol crystals in the VB ↑ with age, also associated with liquification of the VB. ***see also Asteroid Hyalosis***

Synechia (SIN-ek-ee-uh) adhesion of the iris to the cornea or the lens

Syneresis (SIN-er-rees-sis) degenerative shrinkage of the VB - may cause retinal detachment

Synergist muscle which augments the action of the primary mover

Synkinesis duel action of muscles associated with each other *wrt eyes* sneezing & blinking simultaneously

Synophrys a single eyebrow going across the forehead

T

Tarsorraphy (TARS-oh-raf-ee) a surgical procedure uniting the upper & lower EL margins

Tarsus AKA Tarsal plates thick CT plates which give structure to the eye, & allows free movement of the EL over the EB, while supporting SLP eyelid muscle. The upper plate is wider & stronger than the lower - any interruption in these structures compromises the EL closure, and may cause corneal drying

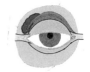

Tectal midbrain syndrome *see Dorsal midbrain syndrome*

Teichopsia (ti-KAP-see-uh) scintillating aura which accompanies a migraine

Telangectasis (tee-lan-jek-TAY-sis) abnormal dilatation of localized capillaries

Telecanthus abnormal intercanthal space but normal interpupillary space

Temporal refers to time & the fact that grey hair (marking the passage of time) often appears first at the site of the temporal bone from the consideration of wisdom in the temple

Temporal arteritis AKA Cranial arteritis

Temporal loop AKA Meyer's temporal loop portion of the optic radiation which is in the temporal lobe of the brain & circles which surround the lateral ventricles

Temporal pallour loss of pinkish colour on the temporal side of the OD, indicative of damage to the ON

Tendon a tie or cord of collagen fibres connecting muscle with bone or *wrt eyes* the EOM to the sclera CT

Tenectomy *wrt eyes* partial or full cutting of a tendon in the eye to reduce or change the power of the EOM

Tenon's capsule *see Fascia bulbi*

Tensor to stretch - generally referring to the action of a muscle which pulls something tighter

Terrien's ulcer thinning of the cornea at the limbus sometimes with vascularization & fat deposits - assoc with progressive astigmatism

Terson's syndrome Hgs in the retina & VB caused by ↑IOP 2° to ↑ intracranial pressure which will clear spontaneously

Thixotropy property of certain gels which can move from liquid to solid on settling & to liquid again on shaking

Thrombus (i) attached intravascular blood clot

Tonic pupil *see Adie's pupil*

Tonometer instrument for measuring IOP either **applanation** - actual pressure on the cornea flattening it slighly & measuring the required P, or **pneumatic** - where a puff of air towards the cornea measures the same thing but the cornea is not touched. P on the EB directly with a finger in a good diagnostician can also provide an estimate - **digital**

Topical application of a substance to the surface of a tissue or structure (≠ **Systemic**)

Torsion rotation around Fick's Y axis (front to back of the eye) so the eye points inwards & outwards *see also Cycloduction*

Torticollis twisted neck resulting in abnormal head position may be related to EOM abnormality &/or spine abnormality

Tortuous twisted, convoluted

Trabeculum AKA Trabecular meshwork *wrt eye* the fibrous network b/n the cornea & iris which drains the AH

Trachoma (TRAK-oh-mar) a serious form of Chlamydial In, in the eye

Transient ischaemic attacks (TIA) mini-strokes, temporary interruption of the BVs with small thrombi which have broken off, moved & lodged in smaller more distal BVs - generally resolves but may leave permanent damage - *wrt eyes* assoc with transient sudden visual changes which resolve over hours & days

Transient Obscuration of Vision temporary VL when standing or sneezing which resolves assoc with ↑IOP &/or ↑intracranial P

Transverse to go across

Transverse axis AKA X axis of Fick plane through the eye around which up & down movements occur

Trichiasis (TRIK-ĭ-a-sis) inversion & rubbing of the ELs against the EB / ingrown ELs / misdirection of the ELs *see also Entropion*

Tritan distrubance in blue perception

Tritanopia inability to see blue

Trochlea (TROK-lee-uh) pulley *wrt eyes* the small cartilaginous loop on the nasal surface of the Frontal bone (upper orbital rim) through which the tendon of the SO moves to direct the EB movement

Tropias divergence of gaze, where the focus on one fovea is not the same as the focus on the other *see also Strabismus*

-tropia *in the eye* an evident or manifest change in eye eg types of squints….*see also - phoria which is only the tendency of an eye to show a change & which may not result in changes to the VA*

True image in diplopia the image derived from the non-deviating eye (≠ **Virtual image**)

Tuberosity (TOOB-er-os-it-ee) a large rounded process or eminence, a swelling or large rough prominence often associated with a tendon or ligament attachment.

Turbinate a child's spinning top, hence shaped like a top; an old term for the nasal conchae.

Tunica layer

Tunica Fibrosa oculi AKA Sclera

Tunica Nervosa oculi AKA Retina

Tunica Vascular oculi AKA Uvea

Tunica Vascular lentis the BVs supplying the crystalline lens until the 5th foetal month

Tylosis ciliaris thickenIng of the EL margins 2° to chronic blcpharitis

Tyndall effect *see Aqueous flare*

U

Ulcer a break in the surface of the skin or MM with T loss & accompanied by If
    corneal loss of the epithelial epithelium
    marginal catarrhal small loss of corneal
    epi. near the limbus

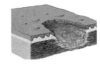

Unharmonious abnormal retinal correspondence AKA Abnormal retinal correspondence adaptation of the retinas to long standing deviation so that a single binocular image is seen from the fovea of the non-deviating eye and the non-fovea but non-corresponding retinal point of the deviated eye merge to form an image *see also harmonious abnormal retinal correspondence, normal retinal correspondence*

Upside-down ptosis lower EL seems higher than the upper EL due to loss of sympathetic innervation *see also Ptosis*

Uvea (YOU-vee-uh) *(Lt –grape)* the vascular layer of the eye = combination of the iris + ciliary body + choroid plexus as a single entity - the BF b/n these 3 structures is continuous and so any pathology tends to involve all 3 at the same time *adj. uveal , uveous*

Uveitis If of one or more portions of the uvea

V

Vacuole (VAK-ew-ohl) small clear intracellular bubble

Varix dilated tortuous BV or lymphatic *adj varicose pl varices*

Veiled glare *see Glare*

Vergance movement of the EBs in opposite directions to maintain a single binocular image

Vernal Conjunctivitis AKA Allergic Conjunctivitis *see Conjunctivitis*

Verruca wart-like *adj verrucous*

Version AKA Conjunctive movement AKA Conjugate movement AKA Gaze movement parallel movement of both eyes in pursuit of an object in any direction

Vertex distance distance from the front of the eye to the back of the glasses lens

Vesicle (VEEZ-ik-el) any membrane enclosed bubble w/n a cell - generally with the same bilipid layered as the CM and so it is possible for the vesicle to generate a separate internal environment w/n the cell - the cell's organelles are forms of vesicles

Vestibulo-ocular reflex AKA Oculo-cephalic reflex involuntary rotation of the eyes in the opposite direction from head rotation to maintain fixation on a non-moving object - abnormal in BStem defects *see also Doll's eyes*

Viral conjunctivitis AKA Pink eye *see Conjunctivitis*

Virtual image image generated by the deviated eye (≠ **True image**)

Visual angle the angle (1) the object subtends on the retina when viewed - expressed as minutes of the visual arc, note the image is actually inverted on the back of the eye, the

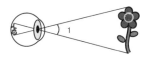

Blind spot subtends < 5° normally - if larger suspect glaucoma

Visual Axis AKA Visual line AKA line of sight AKA Principle line of focus

Visual field (VF) is the area perceived from the vision of one or both eyes - reduction may not be perceived until tested indicating loss of eyesight and its position

> **VF testing** - the extent of the area visible to the eye when it is fixating straight ahead
>
> **Normal Visual Field** depends upon the size & colour of the target, but the monocular range is 60° nasally/ 100° temporally / 60° superiorly / 70° inferiorly, & the binocular range is an oval 200° laterally & 130° vertically. The OD or blind spot is in the Temporal field but cannot be detected in the binocular VF. *see also Blind Spot, Scotomas*

Visual Efficiency the % of loss of VA with each loss of a level of discrimination - also related to the phakic state

Visual Evoked Response AKA Visual Evoked Potential (VEP) computerized recording of activity in the Occipital cortex resulting from retinal stimulation with flashes of light

Visual Pathway (VP) the complete course of the afferent visual input from the retina to the visual brain to the VAA

Visual Perception AKA Eyesight AKA Sight AKA Vision the ability to interpret the surroundings from the visual light hitting the eye; this requires an intact visual system

Visual Preservation AKA Palinopsia

Visual Purple *see Rhodospin*

Visual Snow Syndrome photophobia, persistent after images, which may be generalized or localized and appear like TV static - related to R. Lingual lobe hypermetabolism

Vitamin A deficiency *wrt eyes* *see Keratomalacia*

Vitelliform maculardegeneration AKA Best's disease inherited PRE degeneration affecting the macula which appears as a "yolk" in the macula region which spreads outwards causing permanent VL

Vitrectomy the removal of the vitreous humour - generally if cloudy or mixed with blood - replaced with saline leads to early formation of cataracts and floaters

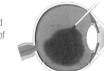

Vitreous *Lt Victrum -glassy* transparent, colourless, gelatinous

Vitreous face condensation of the VB on the back of the EB or immediately post-lental (behind the lens)

Vitreous floaters AKA Floaters moveable opacities in the VB which cast shadows on the retina interfering in VA - considered part of the normal aging process may predict RD if they suddenly increase in numbers &/or size

Vitreous humour a transparent colourless gelatinous mass which fills the EB behind the lens

Vitreous lamina AKA Bruch's membrane a modified glassy thickened BM lying under the RPE *see also Bruch's membrane*

Vitreous opacities any substance in the vitreous gel which interferes with the incident light eg FBs, floaters, Hgs etc. - these may not interfere with VP as they may be compensated for in the binocular VF

Vitreous syneresis shrinkage of the VB ↑ with age & dehydration

Vortex veins AKA Venae Vorticosae the 4 veins (2 superior / 2 inferior) of the EB which provide main venous drainage exiting from the EB at the equator b/n the insertions of the Recti m to the ophthalmic v

Vossius ring pigment fragments from the iris deposited on the front of the lens after blunt trauma - which resolves

W

Wagner's disease hereditary disease of viteoretinal degeneration with retinal tears & detachment, strabismus, myopia & cataracts beginning in the teenage years assoc with Marfan's syndrome

Warped Cornea AKA Pseudokeratoconus temporary corneal distortion due to CLs &/or chalazions

Weigner's lig. AKA Wieger's lig. *see Hyaloideocapsular lig*

Wessely ring small ring on the limbus of the cornea due to the deposits of If cells indicates a reaction to an antigen

White of the eye AKA Sclera

Whitnall's lig transverse suspensory lig from the trochlea to the lacrimal gld - condensing over the SLP & SR to form their muscle sheaths

Word blindness AKA Alexia

Wormian bone extra-sutural bone in the skull

X

Xanthelasma (ZANTH-el-az-muh) fatty deposits in the dermis around the area of the medial canthus associated with DM & hyperlipidaemia

Xanthopsia vision tinted with yellow 2° to drops, digitalis medication jaundice or hysteria

xero (ZAIR-oh)- dry

Xerophthalmia drying of the surfaces of the EB, assoc with Vitamin A deficiency & inability to close the ELs properly

Xerosis (ZER-oh-sis) process of drying the cornea & conjunctiva

Xerostoma dry mouth

Y

Yellow spot AKA Macula lutea

Yoke muscles AKA Contralateral synergists muscles which move the 2 eyes together in the one dimension e.g. L LR & the R MR move both eyes to look left & have equal innervation in each eye (Hering's law of equal innervation).

The 6 cardinal positions of gaze are shown here with their yoke muscle pairs.

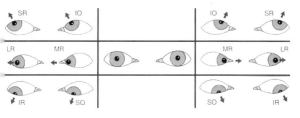

Z

Zonule the numerous fine T strands that stretch across the ciliary processes to the equator of the lens and hold the lens in place. Relaxation allows the lens to curve more & focus on closer objects

Zygomatic N br of CN V$_2$ which innervates the skin below the lower EL & the temporal region

Anterior Chamber

Anteriolateral view

Gonioscopic view

The anterior chamber of the eye is that area directly deep to the cornea and above the iris. It is filled with aqueous humour produced by the CB, and drained by the canal of Schlemm a venous sinus at the base of the cornea.

1   anterior chamber
2   line of Schwalbe - the upper extent of the
3   trabecular meshwork
4   collarette - of the iris
5   ruff - of the iris
6   sinus venous sclerae AKA canal of Schlemm
7   collecting channels
8   cornea
      i = inner surface of
9   pupil
10 iris
11 angle b/n cornea and iris
12 sclera
      s = scleral spur

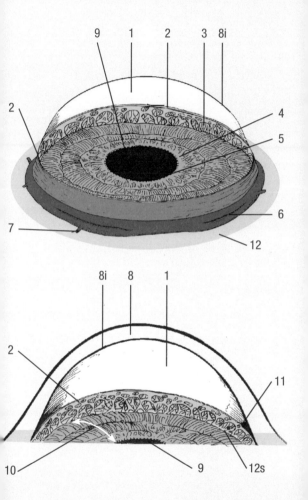

Aqueous humour (AH)

LP showing production and drainage pathway
HP showing major structures of the region of the anterior chamber

The AH is produced by the ciliary epithelium in the post. chamber courses through the to the ant. chamber and is drained mainly via the canal of Schlemm, but also the uveal vessels, (see the purple line). It maintains the IOP at 15-16 mmHg and the shape of the globe & cornea important for the eye's focus and provides nutrition to the cornea, lens & parts of the iris. Blockage of the fluid's drainage will ↑ IOP and cause VL; this is glaucoma.

1   chambers of the eye
      a = anterior
      p = posterior
2   line of Schwalbe
3   trabecular meshwork
4   ruff - of the iris - edge of the pupil
5   lens
6   zonules - ligaments of the lens
7   ciliary processes - produce the AH
8   scleral spur
9   muscles of the CB
10 ant. ciliary v
11 deep & interscleral venous plexi
12 aqueous v
13 canal of Schlemm AKA sinus venosus sclerae
14 cornea
15 iris CT cells
16 posterior epithelium & BM of the iris
17 CB
18 major arterial circle
19 sclera
20 fascial sheath of the EB
21 conjunctiva
22 limbus - junction of sclera & cornea
23 conjunctival limbus

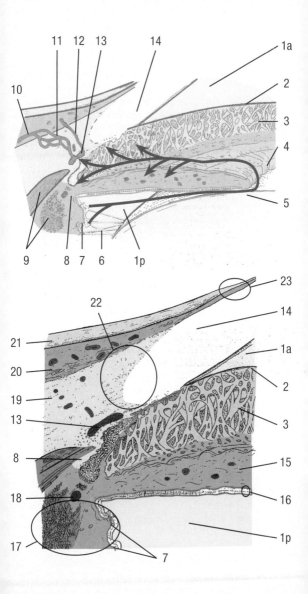

Brodmann's areas

Schema of the cerebral areas related to vision
A lateral surface of the CH
B medial surface of the CH
Frontal lobe
Occipital lobe
Parietal lobe
Temporal lobe

Brodmann areas are areas of the brain where the anatomy &
function & are related. The areas concerned with visual reception
& interpretation are: 17-19, relating images with higher functions
include 20-21. Area 8 (frontal eye fields) is responsible for saccades.

Area	Anatomical location	Name	Function
17	medial surface of the Occipital lobe (+ small lateral extension on the post. pole)	1° visual cortex (V1) AKA Striate cortex	specialized processing of visual input in particular moving & static objects
18 /19 parastriate area	Occcipital lobe (O) - Calcarine sulcus (C)	2° & 3° visual cortex (V2, V3)	Interpretation of shapes, objects and feature recognition
20	inf Temporal gyrus in the Temporal lobe (T)	3° visual cortex (V3)	High level visual processing eg reading
21	middle Temporal gyrus	3° visual cortex (V3) + auditory gyrus	Language recognition & assoc with sounds

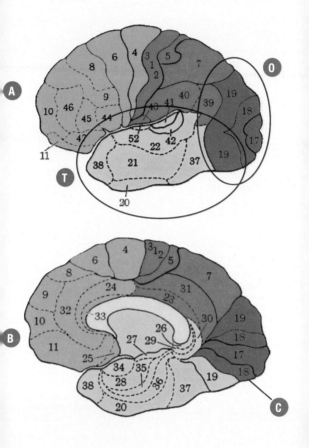

Bruch's membrane AKA Vitreous Lamina

A Schema of normal Bruch's membrane
B Schema of Bruch's membrane with Drusen - Dry Macular Degeneration

Bruch's membrane is a modified clear BM lying underneath the RPE. Nourishment from the choriocapillaris diffuses through the layer and supplies the specialized cells of the retina. Hence any thickening will compromise the BS of the retinal cells.

With ↑ age, ↑ BP & ↑ cholesterol levels other yellow to white deposits may also be found in this layer, called Drusen. While they remain small and trapped in the BM, they have no effect, but as they ↑ in size & number, they affect VA & the health of the retinal cells.

1 retinal special sensory cells
    c = cone cells
    r = rod cells
2 RPE
    d = dead / dying RPE
3 Bruch's membrane
4 Choriocapillaris = capillaries in the choroid
5 Drusen
    L = large deposits thickening the membrane
    s = small deposits trapped in the BM

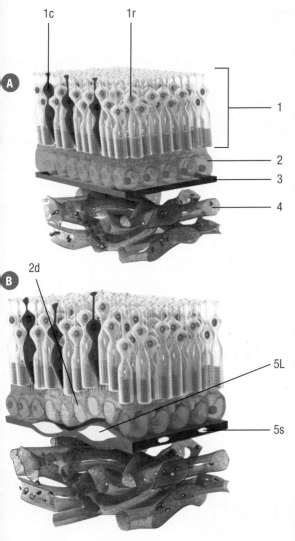

A

1c

1r

1

2

3

4

B

2d

5L

5s

Bruch's membrane AKA Vitreous Lamina AKA Lamina Vitrea

Schema HP

Bruch's membrane is a modified thickened clear basal lamina lying underneath the RPE. It has several layers of fibres, acting as filters and support, which may become thickened with deposits from the diffusion of the capillaries of the choriocapillaris (eg Drusen). If this occurs it will compromise the nutrient flow to the RPE and ends of the special sensory cells of the retina - the rods and cones.

1 endothelium of the choriocapillaris
2 interrupted BM of the choriocapillaris
3 outer collagenous zone
4 elastic layer
5 inner collagenous zone
6 BM of RPE - note invaginations of the BM
7 RPE

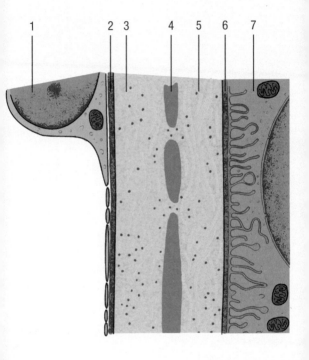

Cavernous venous sinus

Superior view - *looking at the base of the skull*

Coronal view - *looking through the sinus - at the level of the red line*

The cranial venous drainage is via a number of slow flowing venous lakes - or sinuses. These thin-walled amuscular channels receive CSF from arachnoid granulations. The cavernous sinus positioned superior to the sphenoid sinus is intimately related to the arterial & nerve supply of the eye, as well as part of its venous drainage.

1　intercavernous sinus

2　cavernous sinus

3　basilar venous plexus

4　marginal sinus

5　confluence of the cranial venous sinuses

6　sigmoid sinus

7　inferior & superior petrosal sinuses

8　sphenoparietal sinus

9　ophthalmic veins

10　pituitary gld

11　internal carotid a

12　CN II - optic N

13　CN III - oculomotor N

14　CN IV -trochlear N

15　CN V divisions 1 & 2 = ophthalmic N (i) & maxillary N (ii)

16　CN VI - abducens N

17　Temporal lobe

18　sphenoid air sinus

19　nasal cavity

20　Sphenoid b

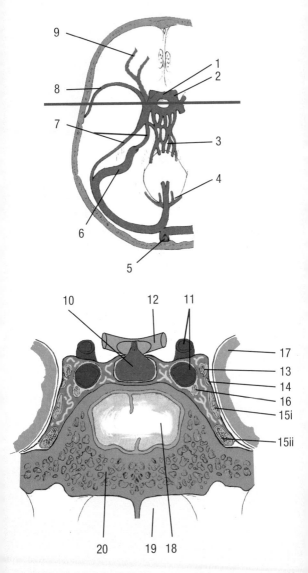

Choroid

Cross-section through the sclera, choroid & RPE
Schema - 3D HP confocal view of the interconnections b/n
the choroid & adjacent layers

The choroid is the vascular layer of the retina, part of the uvea. It is in close proximity to Bruch's membrane through which it supplies the RPE & the specialist sensory ends of the rods & cones, and the deeper layers of the retina.

BF through this vascular T is as follows:
short ciliary a → arterioles → choriocapillaris → venules → vortex v.

1 **suprachoroidea**
2 **large vortex veins**
3 **stroma of the choroid**
4 **choriocapillaris**
5 **Bruch's membrane -**
     5c = collagen layers (upper & lower)
     5e = middle elastica - elastic fibre network in the
           centre of the membrane
6 **RPE**
7 **brush border of the RPE with sensory endings emmeshed**
8 **medium BVs in the choroid stroma**
9 **venules**
10 **short ciliary a**
11 **short ciliary N**
12 **network of N fibres throughout the choroid layers**
13 **stellate melanocytes of the choroid**
14 **sclera**
15 **CT in the sclera**

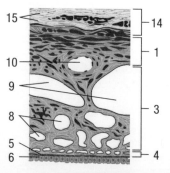

© A. L. Neill

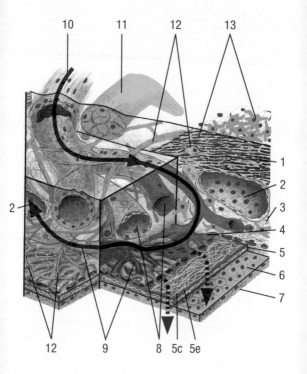

Ciliary Body (CB)
Blood Supply

Sagittal view – cut through the body of the CB & the ring of the iris

The BS of the CB is part of the choroid plexus. The venous drainage is via the canal of Schlemm a venous sinus similar to those found in the CNS, and which also drains the fluid of the ant. chamber. If this drainage is reduced or blocked the IOP will pathologically increase and glaucoma may develop, with irreversible loss of vision.

1 cornea
2 anterior chamber
3 canal of Schlemm
4 iris
5 CB
6 major arterial circle of the iris
7 long post. ciliary a
8 ant. ciliary a & v
9 conjunctival plexus
10 bulbar conjunctiva
11 conjunctival capillary loops
12 corneal epithelium

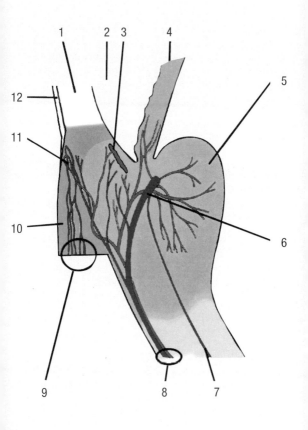

Ciliary Body (CB)
Muscles

transverse view – cut through the ring of structures

The CB is intimately related to the choroid & iris. The processes hold the lens in place, and the muscles control the aperture of the pupil, and curvature of the lens. The ciliary epithelium produces the fluid for the anterior chamber.

1. cornea
2. corneo-scleral junction – limbus
3. sclera
4. longitudinal m – AKA meridional m – responsible for opening the pupil aperture
   Dilator Pupillae m
5. oblique radial muscle fibres of the CB - responsible for the tension on the Zonular fibres and lens
6. circular m AKA Constrictor Pupillae - closes the pupil and inhibits fluid drainage
7. ciliary body processes – site of attachment of the zonules & production of fluid for the ant. chamber
8. iris
9. anterior chamber
10. trabecular network - when open fluid drainage is facilitated
11. canal of Schlemm – venous sinus draining the area of blood & fluid

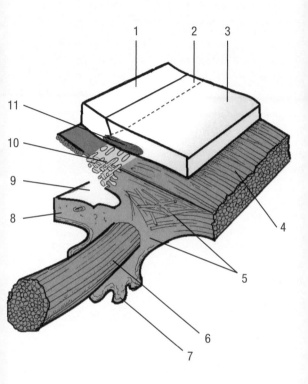

Conjunctiva

Schema

The conjunctiva is a thin stratified epithelial covered fascial layer which lines the inside of the ELs and covers the sclera. It is continuous with the avascular epithelium of the cornea. It contains BVs which supply these structures. Goblet cells facilitate the smooth blinking of the eye, by supplying mucous & oil and the resident T & B cells provide immune protection. If irritated the CT layer thickens and the BVs ↑ forming a pterygium which may grow and encroach upon the cornea.

A   bulbar conjunctiva (on the EB)
B   fornix of the conjunctiva (corners of EB)
C   palpebral conjunctiva (on the EL)

1   fornix
2   palpebral conjunctiva CT layer containing resident immune cells
3   sebaceous & mucous glds
4   stratified epithelium of the palpebral conjunctiva containing goblet cells
5   tarsal plate
6   stratified epithelium of the cornea w/o an underlying CT layer
7   junction b/n corneal & conjunctival epithelium
8   bulbar conjunctiva
9   "grey line" demarkation b/n inner mm and outer skin of the EL

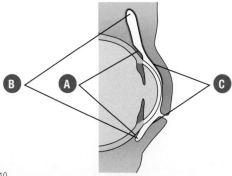

© A. L. Neill

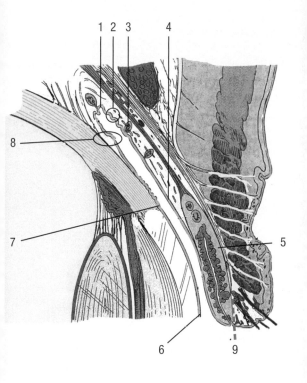

Cornea
Structure

A - epithelium + upper stroma
B - endothelium + Descemet's membrane + deepest
*   stromal layers*
C - stroma - fibroblasts + collagen layers
D - NS of the cornea

These views are of the central cornea. There are 3 merging layers: the surface stratified epi. which changes from rounded basal cells to flattened - "wing cells" joined together tightly to secure the surface & maintain the tear film, (this epi. turns over every 7 days); the largest middle CT stroma of empty fibrocytes & collagen layers in a strict lattice formation (90% of the cornea) and the deep thin flattened endothelium which faces the interior of the ant. chamber. The cornea makes up 2/3 of the EB's RP.

1   epithelium
      b = basal cells - site of new epithelial layers
      t = tight junctions
      L = lymphocyte in basal layer
      m = microvilli
      t = tight junctions
      w = wing cells

2   BM of the surface epithelium
      2b = Bowman's membrane a development from the BM

3   corneal N

4   collagen fibres of the stroma -
      in organized lamellae (o) clear
      disorganized cornea (d) cloudy
      D = collagen fibres in Descemet's membrane

5   stroma
      k = keratocytes/fibrocytes
      m = macula occludans b/n the cells - only in the
         corneal fibrocytes

6   Descemet's membrane

7   BM of the endothelium

8   endothelium

9   marginal projections & folds b/n the endo cells also
     containing cell to cell adhesions

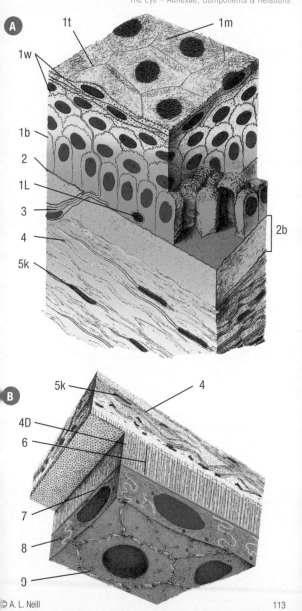

A

1t

1m

1w

1b

2

1L

3

4

5k

2b

B

5k

4

4D

6

7

8

9

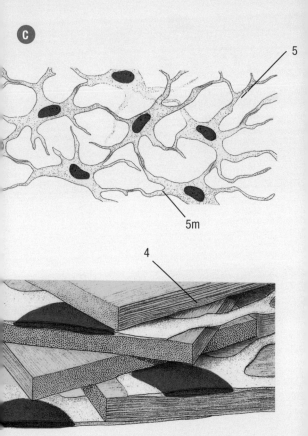

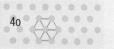

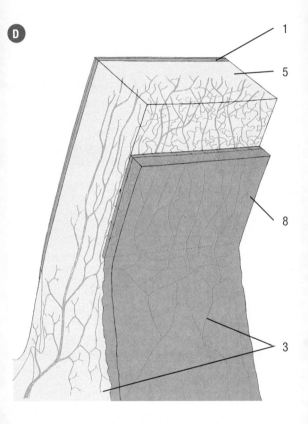

D

1

5

8

3

Cornea
Development

A - 5-6 weeks
B - 7-8 weeks
C - 12 weeks
D - 20 weeks
E - 7 months - developed adult structure

These views are of the central part of the cornea – and do not show the limbus. After 7 months the adult form of the cornea is established. It continues to grow, organize the keratocytes and their collagen fibres until it is filled with densely packed parallel collagen fibres dispersed with thin highly orientated empty cells & their nuclei. The surface epithelium forms flattened surface cells - wing cells which keep the cornea hydrated. With age the turnover of the epithelium ↓ but the surface cells continue to slough, causing "dry eye".

1 epithelium – 2 layers
    b = basal cells - site of new epithelial layers
    w = wing cells, small flattened surface epithelial
        cells which support the thin fluid film & keep the
        cornea hydrated and smooth
2 BM of the surface epithelium
    2b = Bowman's membrane a development from the BM
3 cellular space separating the epithelium & epithelium and
   their BMs invaded by the mesodermal cells
4 BM of the endothelium
    4d = Descemet's membrane a development from the BM
5 mesenchyme moving in from the periphery changing into
    f = fibroblasts and forming
    k = keratocytes which form the ...
    s = stroma of the cornea
6 endothelium
7 keratocytes
    d = disorganized keratocytes in the superficial region of
        the cornea
    p = parallel mature organized keratocytes
8 collagen fibres
    d = thicker disorganized fibres
    m = mature thin parallel fibres

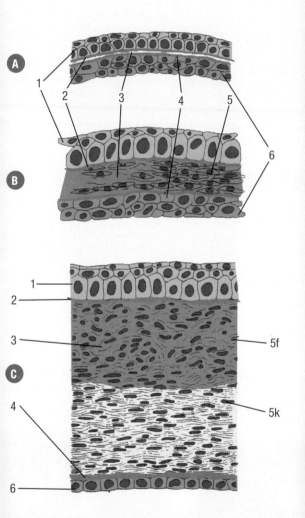

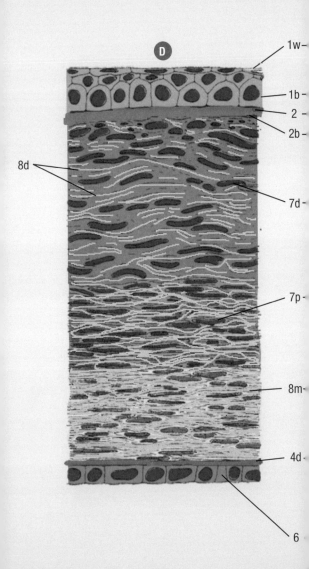

D

1w–
1b –
2 –
2b–

8d

7d–

7p –

8m–

4d –

6

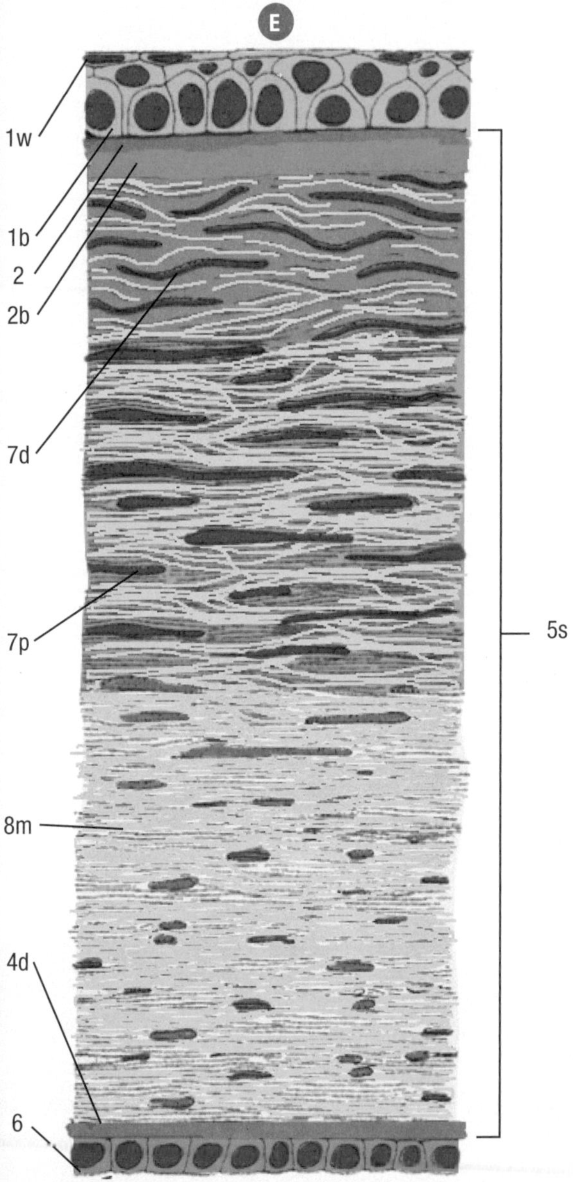

1w

1b

2

2b

7d

7p

5s

8m

4d

6

© A. L. Neill

Crystalline Lens AKA Lens

Schema - lateral views
the lens w/o its capsule
the capsule - showing thickenings
the lens showing changes in the nucleus

The lens is suspended b/n the iris and the VB and held in place by the zonules of the CB, which attach to the capsule along the anatomic equator and contract to decrease its curvature and allow for focus of more distant objects. With relaxation the fibres allow the lens to spring back to the more convex shape which focuses on closer objects. This recoil reduces with age, compromising the ability to focus on near objects. The refractive ability of the lens is about 18 dioptres ~1/3 of the total refractive power of the EB. The cornea makes up the other 2/3.

A = Anterior Pole

E = Equatorial Plane / equator of the lens

P = Posterior Pole

d = depth 4mm / h = height - or diameter 10mm - these vary with focus & age

1 capsule note the thickened areas of the anterior & posterior sections in order to mould the shape of the lens - similar in composition to the BM

2 lens epithelium - cuboidal cells down the anterior surface

3 cortex - which is very felxible and "fluids" in youth decreasing with age

4 nuclei - which harden & increase with age

a = adult

f = foetal

e = embryonic

5 lens fibres - tightly packed cells growing down the lens length in concentric circles

6 germinal zone with columnar germinal epithelium - source of fibres and anterior lens epithelial cells

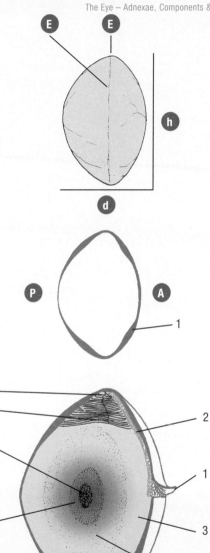

Crystalline Lens AKA Lens

Development

The lens begins as a placode, a differentiating optic cup starts to invaginate.

A = lens placode

B = formation of lens vesicle

C = ant. & post. epithelial layers on either side of the vesicle

D = elongation of the post. epithelial layer to form primary lens fibres - at this stage fat full cells with multiple organelles.

E = ant. cuboidal epithelium / post. fibre layer - progressively fill the lens vesicle completely forming the embryonic nucleus & the ant. & posterior bow sutures - note the forward movement of the nuclei as the fibres elongate

F = optic cup is invaded by mesenchyme and the hyaloid a deteriorates as the lens fibres elongate

G = optic cavity is formed as the lens vesicle is filled and the ELs are separated

1   developing upper EL

2   corneal epithelium

3   ant. epithelium of the lens

4   nuclei of posterior layer in the lens

5   mesenchyme invading the optic cup

6   RPE

7   neural layers of the retina

8   VB

9   remanent of the hyaloid a which connected the back of the eye to the lens - site of floaters ↑ age

10 intraretinal space

11 ant. chamber

12 ora serrata

A

B

C

D

E

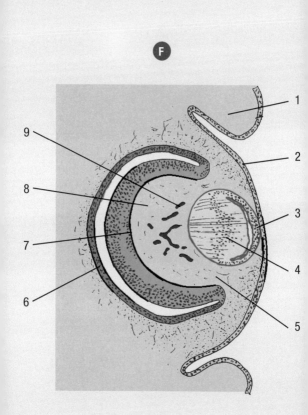

F

© A. L. Neill

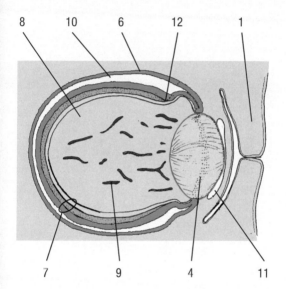

G

Crystalline Lens - Lens

Fibres

The lens is made up of a series of fibrous concentric circles progressively laid down from the germinal zone in the equatorial plane. The lens Y-shaped bow is on the anterior surface and fibres beginning on the arms of the Y will end on its spoke. With age more lens fibres are laid down and they become progressively tighter, thinner and emptier - devoid of organelles. They also harden with age so that when released from the zonules they do not bounce back and become rounder, hence they are less able to focus on near objects. Nearly all elasticity of the lens is lost by 60 yo.

A = lens

B = lens fibre suture pattern - foetal nucleus

C = lens fibre suture pattern - adult lens cortex

1   germinal zone on equatorial plane
2   laying down new epithelium and fibres
3   capsule - basal lamina of the lens
4   growing fibre deposition
5   lens epithelium - cuboidal cells down the anterior surface
6   cortex - site of nuclei of lens cells
7   anterior fibre suture
8   posterior fibre suture

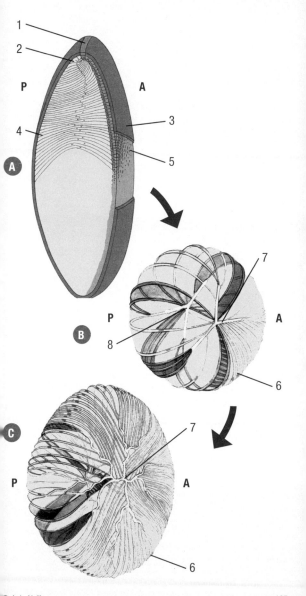

1
2

P   A

4

A

3

5

P   A

B

7

8

6

C

P   A

7

6

Eye
Blood Supply - arterial

Schema - superior view
looking down onto the R eye socket

Branches of the ophthalmic a supply the eye and its adnexae.

1 dorsonasal a
2 medial palpebral a
3 supraorbital a
4 Frontal bone
5 lacrimal gld
6 long post. cilial a
7 zygomatico-temporal & facial a
8 short post. cilial a
9 recurrent meningeal a
10 central retinal a
11 Lateral Rectus m
12 lacrimal a
13 ophthalmic a
14 external carotid a
15 ON = CN II
16 Medial Rectus m
17 ethmoidal sinus with ant & post ethmoidal a
18 trochlea
19 Superior Rectus m
20 supratrochlear a

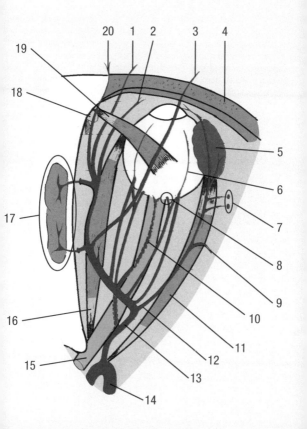

Eye
Blood Supply
Algorithm of arterial supply

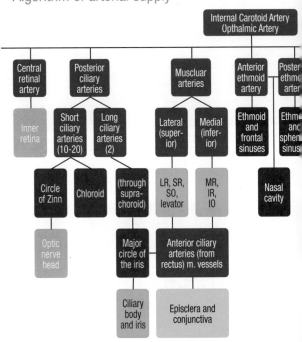

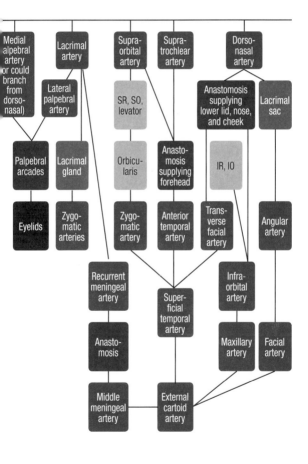

Eye
Blood Supply - venous

Schema - lateral view

looking onto lateral wall of the R eye socket

Branches of the ophthalmic v drain the eye and its adnexae.

1 frontal sinus
2 supraorbital v
3 inferior ophthalmic v
4 facial v
5 Maxilla
6 maxillary sinus
7 pterygoid venous plexus
8 maxillary v
9 cavernous sinus
10 lacrimal v
11 long ciliary v
12 superior ophthalmic v
13 vorticose v (1 of 4 around the EB)

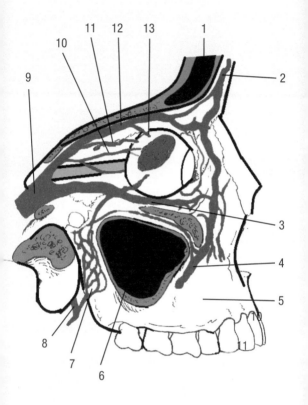

Eye
Nerve supply - Autonomic

Parasympathetic NS of the eye

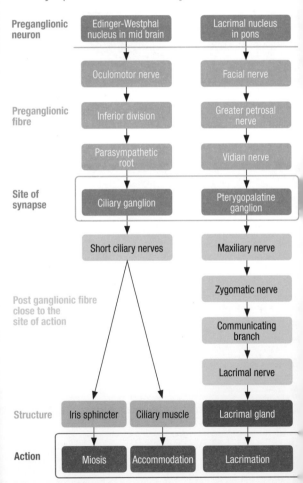

Preganglionic neuron	Edinger-Westphal nucleus in mid brain	Lacrimal nucleus in pons
	Oculomotor nerve	Facial nerve
Preganglionic fibre	Inferior division	Greater petrosal nerve
	Parasympathetic root	Vidian nerve
Site of synapse	Ciliary ganglion	Pterygopalatine ganglion
	Short ciliary nerves	Maxiliary nerve
		Zygomatic nerve
Post ganglionic fibre close to the site of action		Communicating branch
		Lacrimal nerve
Structure	Iris sphincter / Ciliary muscle	Lacrimal gland
Action	Miosis / Accommodation	Lacrimation

© A. L. Neil

Sympathetic NS to the eye

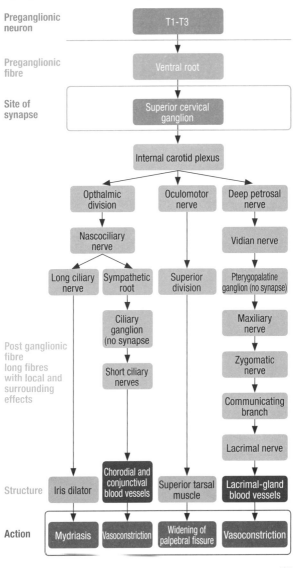

Preganglionic neuron		T1-T3	
Preganglionic fibre		Ventral root	
Site of synapse		Superior cervical ganglion	

Internal carotid plexus

Opthalmic division	Oculomotor nerve	Deep petrosal nerve
Nascociliary nerve		Vidian nerve

Long ciliary nerve	Sympathetic root	Superior division	Pterygopalatine ganglion (no synapse)
	Ciliary ganglion (no synapse		Maxiliary nerve
	Short ciliary nerves		Zygomatic nerve
			Communicating branch
			Lacrimal nerve

Post ganglionic fibre long fibres with local and surrounding effects

Structure	Iris dilator	Chorodial and conjunctival blood vessels	Superior tarsal muscle	Lacrimal-gland blood vessels
Action	Mydriasis	Vasoconstriction	Widening of palpebral fissure	Vasoconstriction

© A. L. Neill

135

Eye
Nerve Supply - overview

Coronal view - muscular base of the eye socket - EB removed
Coronal view - apex of the orbit

CNs III, IV & VI control the movement of the EB: the SO is controlled by CN IV = the trochlear N; the LR is controlled by CN VI = the abducens N & the oculomotor N = CN III, controls the rest.

CN II = the optic N is the special sensory CN for vision, and the CN V1 = the ophthalmic N is the sensory supply of the EB and its adnexae.

1 recti muscles 4 in the eyes i = inferior / L = lateral / m = medial / s = superior

2 CN II

3 CN III s = superior div. g = ciliary ganglion / i = inferior div.

4 CN IV

5 opthalmic vein i = inferior / s = superior

6 CN VI

7 frontal N - branch of CN V_1

8 nasociliary N - branch of CN V_1

9 optic canal

10 ophthalmic a

11 CTR

12 lacrimal N - branch of CN V_1

13 Oblique muscles i = inferior / s = superior

14 Levator palpabrae superioris

15 superior orbital fissure - exit in the orbital cavity for the CNs & BVs

16 Trochlea - ligamentous ring for superior oblique

17 orbital cavity

18 supraorbital notch

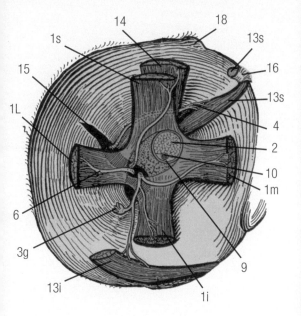

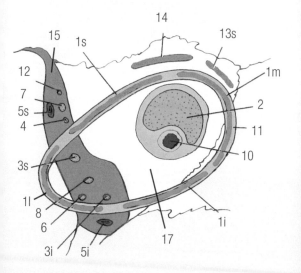

Eye
Nerve Supply - overview

Superior view - deep (D) & superficial (S)
Looking down onto the ACF

CNs III, IV & VI control the movement of the EB: the SO is controlled by
CN IV = the trochlear N; the LR is controlled by CN VI = the abducens
N & the oculomotor N = CN III, controls the rest, including the tarsal
muscles of the EL. CN II = the optic N is the special sensory CN for
vision, and the CN V_1 = the ophthalmic N is the sensory supply of
the EB & its adnexae, including the lacrimal gld. CN VII = facial N
innervates the ELs & Orbiularis oculi m so trauma will result in an
open weeping eye, but a permanently ptosed eye of gradual onset is
often due to damage to CN III.

1   **EB**
- r = retina
- s = sclera

2   **ON** → optic chiasm → optic tract

3   **CN III** = oculomotor N

4   **CN IV** = trochlear N & its muscle SO
- i = infratrochlear br

5   **CN V** = trigeminal N at the site of the ganglion and
formation of the 3 divisions
- i = CN V1= ophthalmic N
- ii = CN V2 = maxillary N
- iii = CN V3 = mandibular N

6   **CN VI** = abducens N & its muscle LR

7   **Levator Palpabrae Superioris m overlying SR**

8   **lacrimal gland & its N**

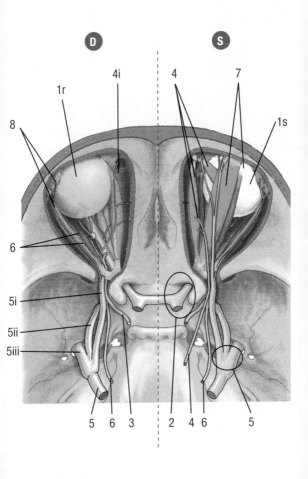

Eye
Nerve Supply - Afferent (Sensory)

ophthalmic N
Schema - superior view
looking down onto the R eye socket

Branches of the ophthalmic N (CN V$_1$), upper division of the Trigeminal N = CN V$_1$ is the afferent (sensory) supply the eye and its adnexae. Fibres of the PaNS travel with these Ns synapse in the ciliary ganglion and innervate the pupillary m.

1   supratrochlear N
2   supraorbital N
3   lacrimal gld & N
4   zygomatico-temporal & facial N
5   short ciliary Ns
6   ciliary ganglion (3 fibre types travel through this ganglion, sym motor Ns, sensory Ns & PaNs)
7   zygomatic N
8   maxillary N (CN V$_2$)
9   trigeminal ganglion of the trigeminal N = CN V
10 ON (CN II)
11 frontal N
12 ethmoid sinus with ant. & post. ethmoid Ns
13 long ciliary N
14 trochlea
15 Superior Oblique m
16 nasociliary N → infratrochear N

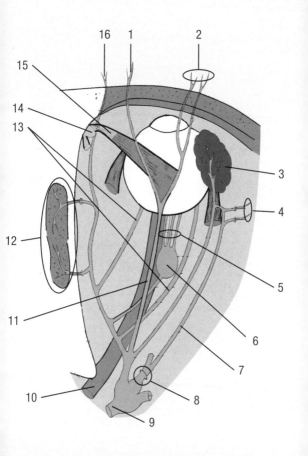

Eye
Supportive Structures

Connective Tissue system & Fascial layers
Coronal views – anterior section of the orbit
looking onto the front of the orbit (A) & mid orbit (B)

In the eye there is considerable connection b/n the muscles and the bony orbit – this helps to stabilize and limit the muscle movement of the muscle cone, guarantee the BS to the eye and permit slight changes in the contents w/o compromising the movements of the EB. With trauma there can be scarring resulting in severe limitation of movement.

1 lacrimal v – with N
2 lacrimal gld
3 periorbita – fascial sheath
4 lateral retinaculum –
   part of the lateral rectus fascial system (s)
5 Inf. Rectus m & br of CN III encased in the inferior rectus fascial system
6 fascia bulbi – thin fascia encasing the EB from the limbus through the mu cone
7 medial rectus fascial system – stronger than the lateral system – to prevent over-abduction in eye movements
8 superior orbital fascial system
9 superior oblique tendon
10 Whitnall's lig
11 Superior Oblique m
12 muscle cone / removed EB
13 frontal N
14 superior rectus-levator fascial system
15 zygomatic N
16 zygomatico-facial N
17 ophthalmic a & v
18 superior ophthalmic v
19 ON with central retinal BVs

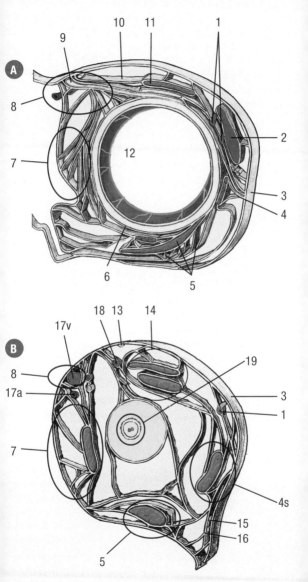

Eye
Supportive Structures

Connective Tissue system & Fascial layers
Sagittal view - through the vertical meridian of the eye -
looking onto the side of the eye in the orbit

In the eye there is considerable connection b/n the muscles and the bony orbit – this helps to; stabilize and limit the muscle movement of the muscle cone, guarantee the BS to the eye and permit slight changes in the contents w/o compromising the movements of the EB. With trauma there can be scarring in these regions resulting in severe limitation of movement and causing adherence syndromes. Note the check ligaments (7) which prevent over activity of the Recti.

1   tarsal plate of the lower EL
2   conjunctiva
3   orbital septum
4   Orbicularis Oculi m
5   subcut. fat
6   periorbita – fascial sheath
7   check ligs
       i = check lig of the IR
       s = check lig of the SR
8   IO
9   inferior rectus facial system
10   falciform lig.
11   Inf. Rectus m + CT sheath
12   ON
13   SR + Levator Palpebrae m + their CT sheaths
14   superior rectus-levator fascial system + levator aponeurosis
15   Müller's m + tarsal plate of the upper EL
16   Tenon's capsule – thin fascia encasing the EB from the limbus through the mu cone - fascia bulbi

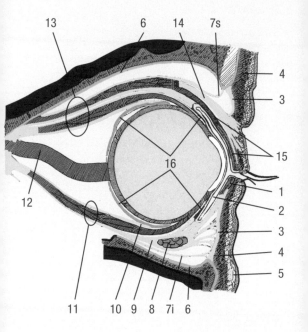

Eye
Supportive Structures

Connective Tissue system & Fascial layers
Transverse view - just above the horizontal/equatorial plane
of the eye (in the UL) in the primary position (normal position
with the ELs closed)

In the eye there is considerable connection b/n the muscles and the bony orbit – this helps to; stabilize and limit the muscle movement of the muscle cone, guarantee the BS to the eye and permit slight changes in the contents w/o compromising the movements of the EB. With trauma there can be scarring in these regions and severe limitation of movement may result from the developing scar tissue.

1 Orbicularis Oculi m
2 superior tarsal plate
3 orbital septum
4 check lig of the LR - part of the lateral fascial CT system
5 periorbita
6 LR + sheath
7 periorbital fat in the muscle cone
8 ON
9 MR
10 ethmoid sinus cell
11 check lig of the MR (stronger than the lateral check lig)
12 lacrimal duct
13 medial palpebral lig with ant. & post. limbs
14 fascia bulbi
15 conjunctiva palpebral (p) & bulbar (b)

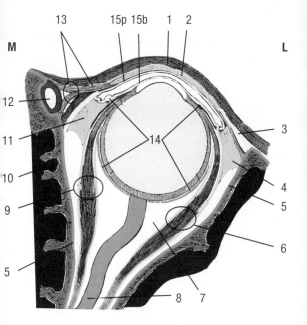

M

L

13   15p 15b   1   2

12

11

10

9

5

14

3

4

5

6

8   7

Eye

External view of the eye and its components

Anterior View - sulci increase with age

Eversion of the Lower Lid - can examine the conjunctiva & assess anaemia

Eversion of the Upper Lid - exposures the upper tarsal plate - cartilaginous support for the lid - & tarsal glands in allergies, & foreign bodies.

1   eyebrow
2   upper eyelid orbital part
3   palpebral sulcus i = inferior, s = superior
4   upper eyelid tarsal part
5   angle of the eye L = lateral m = medial in b/n the palpebral fissure 5f (where the upper & lower lids meet)
6   nasal jugal sulcus
7   eyelashes
8   malar sulcus = lateral sulcus
9   iris
10 pupil
11 sclera = bulbar conjunctiva
12 papilla lacrimalis (raised surface)
13 punctum lacrimale (opening for tear duct)
14c caruncula lacrimalis = lacrimal caruncle - (tear duct)
14s sac for lacrimal gland
15 lacus lacrimalis
16 plica semilunaris
17 palpebral conjunctiva
18 lower lid margins (ant & post)
19 tarsal glands and openings
20 inf fornix of the conjunctiva
21 branches of posterior conjunctival arteries
22 tarsal plate (lower is much thinner 22L)
23 upper lid margins (ant & post)

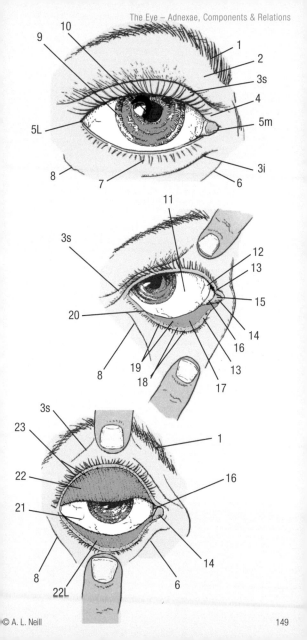

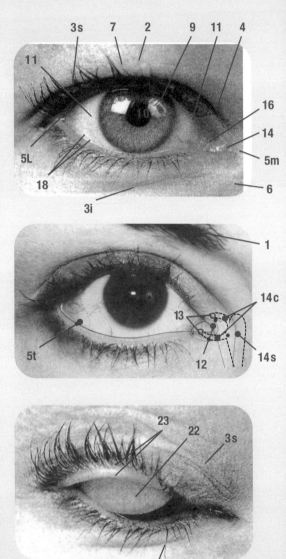

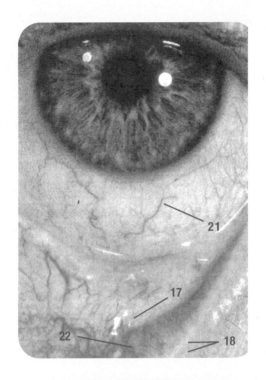

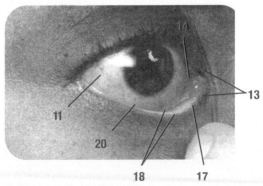

Eyeball (EB)
Anaesthesia

A - ant. view subcutaneous infiltration – also site of peribulbar roof & floor approaches with deeper penetration

B - ant. view of retrobulbar injection – skin – lower EL approach

C – ant. view of retrobulbar injection – conjunctival approach

D – lat. view of retrobulbar injection – into the ciliary ganglion

E – lat. view anterior chamber

Anasthesia is used to paralyse the muscles of the eye for extraocular & introcular procedures such as: correction of strabismus & relocation of muscle insertions, corneal procedures, glaucoma cataract surgery & laser treatment of the cornea.

Four main methods are used:
- subcutaneous infiltration for the surface and superficial facial muscles – to stop blinking and the corneal reflex, this is always undertaken in ocular surgery (A);
- peribulbar injection – a non-specific injection into the roof or onto the floor of the orbit – for non-specific paralysis of extra & intraorbital muscles (A);
- retrobulbar injection into specific muscles or Ns as N blocks (B,C & D)
- and the less commonly used anterior chamber injection specifically for intracular muscles and patient comfort (E)

1 **peribulbar space – around the muscle cone of the orbit**
2 **frontal sinus**
3 **muscle cone – injections into this space may compress the ON & cause ↑ OP. This space is best used for specific N or muscle injection**
4 **maxillary sinus**
5 **ciliary ganglion – providing innervation for the CB muscles**
6 **ON**
7 **ACF**

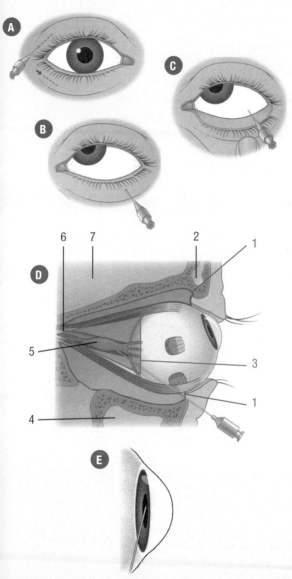

153

Eyeball (EB)
Dimensions

Schema -

A anterior view of the EB

B lateral view of the cornea & limbus

C sagittal section through the EB

The dimension of the lens varies with age and stage. There is also a large normal variation. It continues to grow throughout life thickening and becoming less flexible. The length of the EB may also alter lengthening as the sclera weakens or with ↑ IOP.

1 11mm radius of the cornea AP – smaller due to scleral encroachment (1s)

2 12 mm radius of the cornea laterally -

3 3mm back of the cornea to the anterior surface of the lens – ↑ with keratoconus & glaucoma

4 0.4-0.6mm corneal thickness

5 0.71-0.75 mm scleral thickness – thicker after the limbus (up to 1.0mm)

6 3-5mm thickness of the cornea depending on age and focus

7 8-12 mm diameter of the lens depending on age & focus – responsible for 1/3 of the refractive power of the EB

8 12 mm radius of the sclera

9 8 mm radius of the cornea – greater curvature and RI – 18 diopters responsible for 2/3 of the refraction in the eye

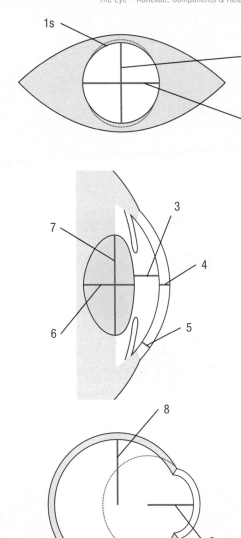

Eyeball (EB)
Blood Supply

Schema -
sagittal view - cut through the eye to view internal layers

The main BS of the orbit and its contents come from the uvea, which is a continuous vascular layer containing the choroid, CB & iris. These are derived from branches of the ophthalmic a, which also supply the extra orbital Ts. Retinal BVs course through the retina at the level of the middle membrane.

1   major circle of the iris
2   iridal arcades
3   lens
4a   ant. chamber
4p   post. chamber
5   anterior ciliary a
6   long post. ciliary a
7   muscular BVs to Lat. Rectus m
8   sclera
9   muscular v
10   retinal BVs
11   choroid BVs
12   vortex v
13   post. ciliary a L= long / s = short
14   central retinal BVs
15   hyaloideo-capsular lig. / Wieger's lig.
16   hyaloid mem.

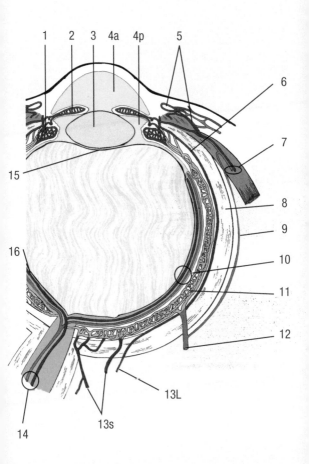

Eyeball (EB)
Blood Supply

Schema - surface views of the EB to show major arterial and venous systems
A lateral view of the EB
B anterior view of the EB
C anterior view of the cornea

The BS of the sclera must also supply the extraorbital muscles, conjunctiva & scleral fascia. The BVs are arranged in anastomotic circles similar to that in the brain. The veins also drain the aqueous humour of the anterior chamber, via a venous sinus as in the cerebrum.

1   minor arterial & venous circles
2   major arterial circle & sinus venous sclerae
3   radial v
4   ant. ciliarly a & v
5   long post. ciliary a + vorticose v
6   short post. ciliary a & v
7   episcleral venous plexus
8   intrascleral venous plexus
9   deep scleral plexus
10 venous collecting channel
11 aqueous v
12 ant. chamber

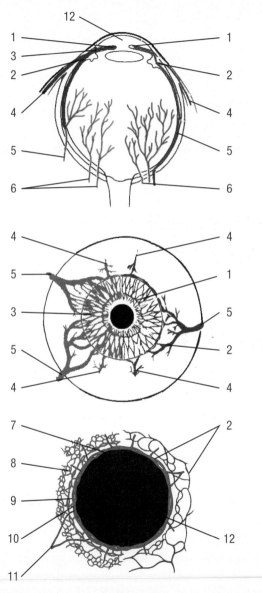

Eyeball (EB)
Layers

Schema

The EB is composed of 3 concentric shells, and divided into 2 connecting spaces.

A   the supporting shell = corneoscleral
B   the vascular shell = the uvea
C   the photosensitive shell = the retina + ON
D   the anterior chamber
E   the posterior chamber

1   sclera
2   cornea
3   meninges
4   tendinous insertions of the extra-ocular muscles
5   CB
6   iris
7   ciliary processes
8   choroid
9   non-visual retina = ora serrata
10 blind spot = emergence of the ON
11 ON
12 fovea - point of sharpest focus
13 RPE
14 retina

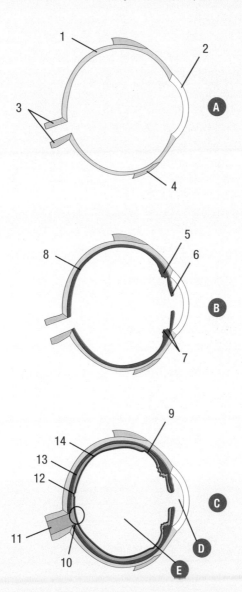

Eyeball (EB)
Shape

Lenses of the eye

The EB is an assembly of a group of "lenses" which work in concert to focus incident light on the retina

1   Vitreous humour = VITREOUS LENS
2   Crystalline lens = LENS
3   Iris controlling the pupillary aperture = LIGHT APERTURE
4   Anterior chamber = AQUEOUS LENS
5   Cornea = COVER LENS
     the main refraction of the light takes place at the cornea

Interaction of EB length, lenses & focus

The interaction b/n the lenses of the eye and the EB length will determine the type of vision possible.

1   Emmetropia - normal vision
2   Hyperopia - focus of parallel light rays falls behind the retina w/o accommodation
3   Manifest hyperopia - accommodation brings the distant object into focus
4   Absolute hyperopia - a corrective lens is needed to focus distant objects
5   Myopia - focus of near objects falls in front of the retina
6   Myopia - focus of distant objects is possible
7   Myopia - a concave corrective lens is needed to focus on near objects

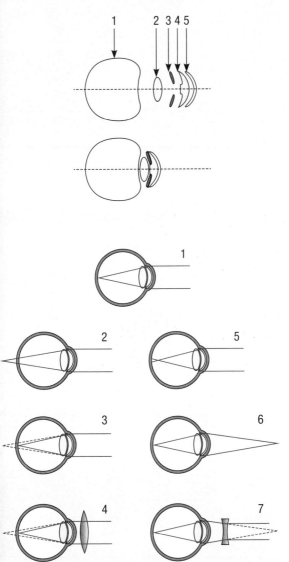

Eyeball (EB)
Structure

Histology
LP H&E overview showing most structures

The EB is the organ of vision. It sits snugly in the eye socket surrounded by loose areolar T to allow for free movement and has a posterior opening to allow for the passage of BVs and the optic N (CN II).

1 cornea

2 pupil

3 anterior (aqueous humour) and posterior chambers of the eye

4 iris

5 ciliary processes from the cilary m

6 suspensory lig = zonular fibres

7 choroid

8 retina

9 optic papilla – blind spot

10 optic N (CN II)

11 macula fovea – focus site

12 vitreous humour – gel like material in the eye should be adherent only at the macula, optic N & ora serrata

13 sclera – white of the eye made of dense CT

14 ora serrata – small section (8mm) of the epithelium b/n the ciliary body and the retina which secretes nutrients into the humours of the eye to supply the internal structures

15 limbus

16 lens

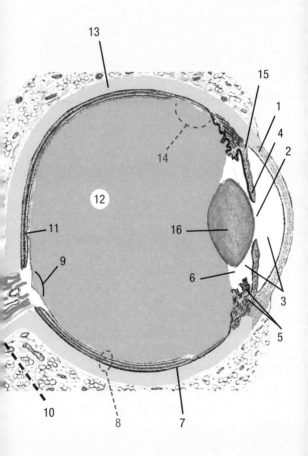

Eyelid (EL)

Histology
LP H&E - overview of most structures

The eyelid protects and facilitates lubrication of the EB. The lamina propria of the subcut. T has a specialist CT dense structure, the tarsi (tarsal plates) which maintain a stiff convex curve as the eyelid moves over the EB surface with blinking.

1 hair follicle
2 adipose cells
3 sebaceous gld of the follicle
4 epidermis
5 sweat glds
6 dermis = CT
7 Orbicularis Oculi m
8 eyelash hair follicles -
9 Ciliary m = muscle of Rollen
10 d = duct / g = gland
11 sweat glds - near eyelashes = glds of Moll
12 tarsus = tarsal plate
13 palpable conjunctiva
14 BVs
15 lymphpoid T
16 superior tarsal muscle = muscle of Muller
17 grey line - demarkation b/n the conjunctiva & skin of the EL

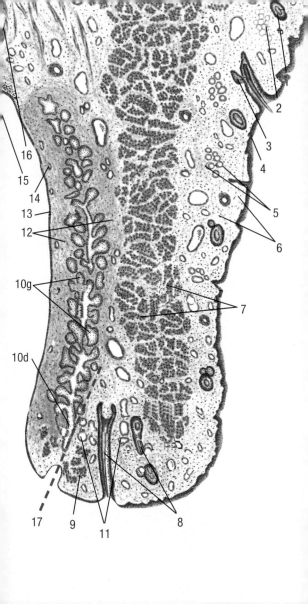

Eyelid (EL)

A anterior view BS arterial
B anterior view NS

The ELs fuses with the retractors & prevents the orbital contents from moving into the subcutaneous T.

1   supratrochlear a + N
2   medial palpebral a i = inferior / s = superior
3   infraorbital a + N
4   marginal arterial arcade i = inferior / s = superior
5   transverse facial a
6   lateral palpebral a i = inferior / s = superior
7   lacrimal a + N
8   peripheral palpebral arcade i = inferior / superior
9   supraorbital a + N
10 infratrochlear N
11 zygomatico-facial N

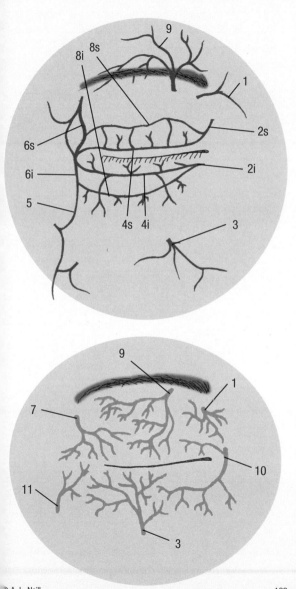

Eyelid (EL)

Muscles & Ligaments
A sagittal view upper EL
B sagittal view lower EL

The ELs wipe over the EB surface closely, lubricating the anterior surfaces, preventing orbital contents from protruding, regulating the light & protecting the EB. The tarsal plates (TP) maintain a convex curve which does not pressure the EB surface. The ELs are closed by OO, (the protractor muscle) and opened by the upper & lower EL retractors

Upper EL retractors : Levator Aponeurosis; Superior Tarsal muscle (Müller's muscle)

Lower EL retractors : Capsulopalpebral fascia; Inferior Tarsal muscle

The orbital septum fuses with the retractors & prevents the orbital contents from moving into the subcut. T.

1 Frontalis m
2 skin of the forehead
3 eyebrow
4 Orbicularis Oculi m
   p = pre-orbital fibres (interdigitate with Frontalis)
   o = orbital fibres around the eye
   s = pre-septal fibres supf to the orbital septum - contraction for normal spontaneous blinking 1/3sec (duration 300ms)
   t = pre-tarsal fibres in the EL -contraction for forced closure of the ELs
5 orbital septum (laxity in the lower EL may result in ectropion)
6 Levator Palpebral Superioris (LPS) m - maintains the resting position of the EL
   a = aponeurosis - expanded insertion tendon
   m = skeletal muscle belly
7 upper EL crease - caused by insertion of LPS aponeurosis into 4t fibres

8 EL skin - thinnest in the body -contains sweat (AKA glands of Moll) & sebum glds & hair follicles
9 TPs containing tarsal glds (AKA Meibomian glds)
10 Inferior Tarsal m
11 peri orbital fat (maintained in position by the septum lower EL fat ↓ may result in entropion)
12 IO
   c = capsulopalpebral fascial head
13 orbital fat
14 IR
15 conjunctiva
   g = conjunctival glands (AKA Krause & Wolfring glands) necessary to maintain the tear film
16 superior peripheral arterial arcade
17 Superior Tarsal m AKA Müller's muscle
18 SO
19 SR

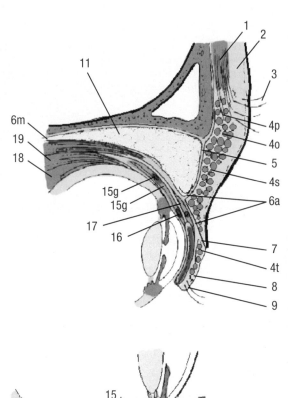

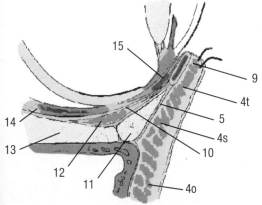

Eyelid (EL)

Muscles BS & NS
A sagittal view - Levator Palpebrae Superioris (LPS) -
retractor
B sagittal view - Orbicularis Oculi (OO) - contractor

The ELs maintain an open position at rest - blinking approx every 3s for 3ms. This is facilitated by LPS and the pretarsal fibres of OO.

Levator Palpebrae Superioris

O   inf aspect of the lesser wing of the Sphenoid - superior to the optic canal

I   superior tarsal plate & skin of the upper EL

A   elevates the EL and maintains it is the open resting position

BS ophthalmic + supraorbital a

NS CN III (oculomotor N) - superior division

Orbicularis Oculi - part of the muscles of facial expression

O   Frontalis, medial margin of the Maxilla, Lacrimal bone

I   inserts into the deep fascia of the orbit on all sides + lateral palpebral raphe

A   tight closure of the ELs & closure of the eyebrows normal blinking by the pretarsal fibres

BS zygomatico-orbital + palpebral brs of the ophthalmic & lacrimal a

NS CN VII (facial N) motor

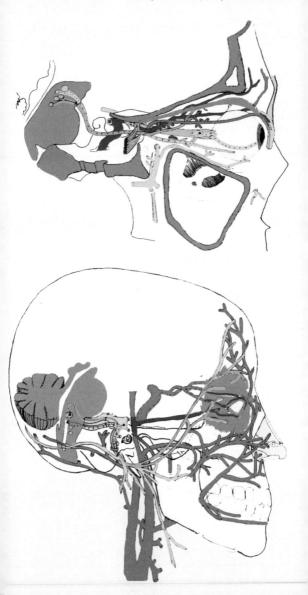

Fovea & Foveola

Histological schema

The foveola is at the centre region of the fovea which the centre of the macula, .5mm in diameter. It is the site of greatest VA. The retinal layers thickest either side of this region (up to 5 ganglion cells thick) in the fovea, again thin in the parafoveal & perifoveal regions, but they are the thinnest in the foveola. They are also avascular in this central region, relying solely upon nutrients diffusing across the Bruch's membrane for nutrition & oxygenation. The cones are smaller hexagonal & densely packed here, with single bipolar cell connections to each cell. Rods appear in the outer regions, and the cones become sparser. Approximately 50% of the visual input comes from the fovea, with the other 50% from the rest of the visual retinal fundus.

L - light pathway

VP - visual response pathway from the retinal layers

1 nerve fibre layer

2 ganglion cells

3 amacrine cells

4 bipolar cells

5 horizontal cells

6 photoreceptors c = cones r = rods

7 RPE

8 Bruch's membrane

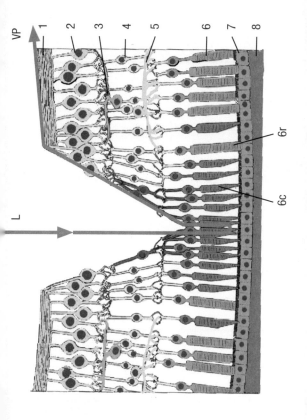

VP

1
2
3
4
5
6
7
8

L

6r

6c

Fundus

view of the normal features of the back of the EB - retina

The integrity of the back of the eye is viewed directly using the ophthalmoscope with or without a dilated pupil

1. OD containing the central retinal BVs – central retinal artey & vein
2. inf nasal retinal v
3. inf temporal retinal a
4. macula
5. fovea
6. superior temporal retinal a
7. superior nasal retinal v

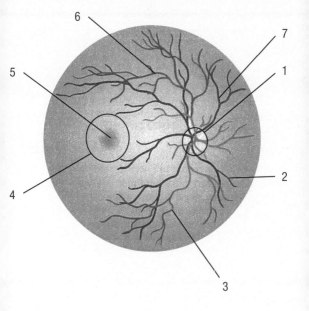

Iris

anterior surface anatomy

The surface anatomy of the iris is highly visible and examination of this region can show early signs of eye disease, when examined correctly. The limbus (or junctional site(s)) has 3 components not clearly visible - the bulbar limbus - site of fusion of the bulbar sheath with the sclera; the corneal limbus site of the corneoscleral junction and the conjunctival limbus - site of the fusion b/n the conjunctiva and the cornea

1 sclera
2 limbus
  b = bulbar limbus
  c = corneal limbus
  co = conjunctival limbus
3 ciliary margin
4 glare - reflection of light on a healthy cornea - can use this reflection to estimate the depth of the anterior chamber
5 pupil
6 pupillary margin
7 contraction furrows
8 Fuch's crypts AKA crypts
9 pigmented stratum

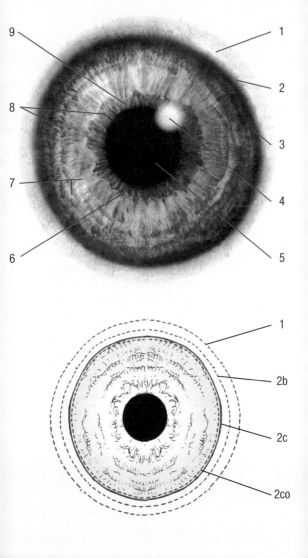

Iris

Schema
anterior overview of layers

The iris has 2 portions - the pupillary (i) & ciliary zones (ii). Its most superficial layer determines the eye colour by the amount of pigment in the melanocytes. The pigment is concentrated at the pupillary opening to absorb scattered & reflected light and improve VA.

Layers superficial to deep

A   anterior limiting layer = pigmented epithelium

B   stromal layer = trabecular layer of collagen & elastin fibre network AKA Blue Iris - w/o melanin this area appears blue in all cases

C   vascular layer - supplied by the long and short ciliary BVs

D   muscular layer = containing the sphincter & dilator ms - which change the diameter of the pupil

E   posterior pigmented epithelium - to further absorb stray light in the EB cavity which is not focused on the retina

1   Fuch's crypts

2   collarette

3   radial contraction furrows

4   pupillary ruff

5   pupillary arcades

6   minor arterial circle

7   iris ms - d = dilator s = pupillary sphincter

8   structural folds of Schwalbe

9   pars plicata of the CB

10 major arterial circle

11 circular contraction furrows

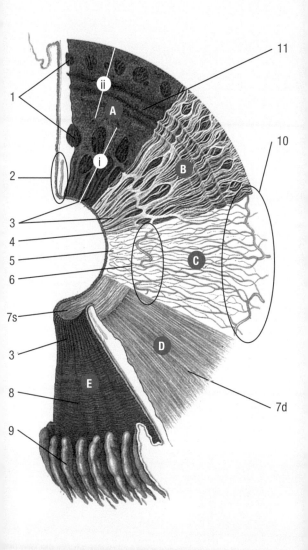

Lacrimal Apparatus (LA) AKA Tears & Tear ducts

Schema - anterior view

The LA consists of the lacrimal glands - small almond shaped glands mainly found in the upper outer corner of each eye socket - the lacrimal fossa, with smaller palpebral parts found along the inside of the eyelid. The ducts to drain their secretions are located in the medial canthus. The glands form tears which may be stimulated by physical or emotional neural input via the ANS. They also lubricate the eye in association with the tarsal glds.

1   **lacrimal gld (main orbital part)**
2   **secretory ducts**
3   **superior (8mm) & inferior (2mm) canaliculi**
4   **common canaliculus**
5   **lacrimal sac (10mm)**
6   **naso-lacrimal duct (12mm)**
7   **inf. nasal concha**
8   **inf. nasal meatus (opening of the duct - bordered by the valve of Hasner)**
9   **nasal cavity**
10   **superior & inferior puncta**

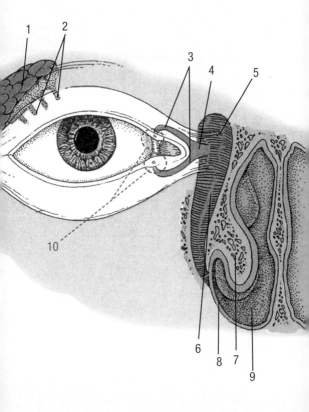

Lacrimal Apparatus AKA Tears & Tear ducts

Histology - MP H&E

This gld lubricates the cornea, via seromucoid secretions. These are essential for corneal health protecting it from dryness & In.

1. myoepithelial cells surrounding the glds
2. adipose cells
3. interlobular excretory duct
4. acini
5. a & v
6. CT septa
7. lacrimal N

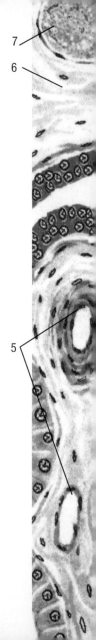

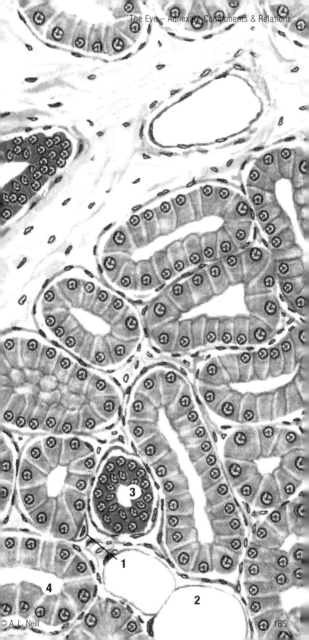

3

1

2

4

Lacrimal gland cell

Schema

The exocrine lacrimal glands secrete a mucino-serous solution which; covers the cornea; prevents dry eyes; protects against infection - via lysozyme an antibacterial enzyme in the lacrimal secretion, and helps to flush out foreign bodies.

Tears are mainly made up of the secretions of the lacrimal cells but there are contributions from the accessory glds, the tarsal glands of the EL and the conjunctival goblet cells.

1   secretory granules
2   basal surface - relatively few granules
3   mitochondria concentrated around the RER in the base
4   RER + free ribosomes
5   nucleolus
6   GA

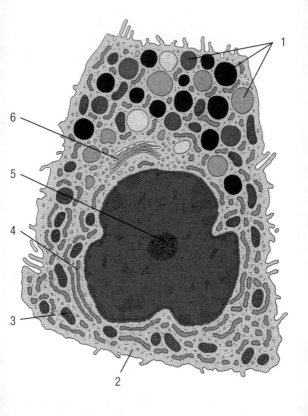

Macula AKA Macula Lutea

Histological schema

The macula represents the area of central vision in the eye. It is bounded by the temporal retinal BV arcades. Eyes will focus an object to this area when "looking". Histologically there are 4 zones which appear as a concavity surrounded by annuli of changing retinal cell layers. Clinically it is visualized as a yellow spot on the retina, due to the deposits of the yellow xanthophyll carotenoids, and its relative avascularity. Within the the fovea (fovea centralis) is the foveola, the area of sharpest focus. It contains a high concentration of cones. On examination - light is reflected from the foveola as a sharp point or high glossy sheen - THE CENTRAL FOVEAL REFLEX.

A foveola - capillary free area >.5mm diameter (retina is the thinnest .13mm)

B fovea ~3.5mm

C parafoveal area / annulus ~.5mm

D perifoveal area / annulus ~1.5mm

A + B + C + D = clinical macula lutea = ~6mm diameter retina thickness ~.18mm

1 VB

2 internal limiting membrane

3 N fibre layer adherent to .....

4 ganglion cell layer -

↑ in the parafoveal annulus up to 7 cells thick changing from 4 to1 cell thick in the perifoveal annulus

5 IPL - note this layer ↓ in the central regions

6 INL - ↑ in the parafoveal annulus up to 12 cells thick

7 OPL note the orientation of the fibres in this area away from the centre causing ↑ retinal thinning in the foveola

8 ONL

9 external limiting layer

10 photoreceptor layer

11 RPE

12 OD site of the ON and emergence of the central retinal BVs

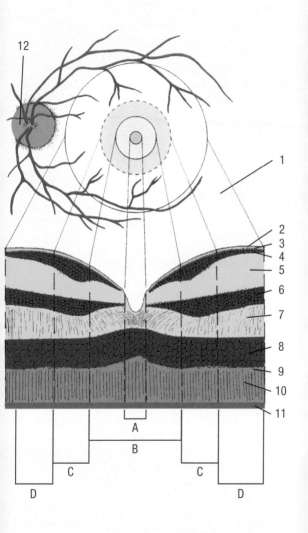

Muscles of the Eye
Lateral view

Extra-ocular muscles - EOM control the gaze and direction of the EB. They move "in concert" and are attached to the sclera of the EB in a spiral. Included in this is the muscle responsible for elevating the EL with changes in the EB gaze.

1 Levator Palpebrae Superioris m - opens the EL
   NS oculomotor N = CN III / supraorbital N - from the Ophthalmic N (CN V$_1$)

2 Recti m - these 4 muscles control the movement of the EB directly
   i = inferior / s = superior
   L = lateral / m = medial
   NS oculomotor N = CN III except for lat. Rectus m - abducent N = CN VI

3 Oblique m - these 2 muscles are attached to the orbit wall via a trochlea (pulley) (3t) & so move the EB in diagonal directions
   i = inferior / s = superior
   NS oculomotor N = CN III except for So - trochlear N = CN IV
   BS ophthalmic a (br of the internal carotid)

4 sclera

5 CTR - site from which all the EOM attach

6 ocular cavity

7 iris

8 optic N = CN II responsible for vision

9 lens

Intra-ocular muscles - IOM control the focus by moving the structures w/n the EB.

10 Ciliaris - which contracts to reduce the curvature of the lens and allow for far sight

11 Dilator pupillae

12 Sphincter pupillae
   NS oculomotor N = CN III + ANS - mainly parasympathetic

13 cornea

14 CB

15 zonula fibres

© A. L. Neill

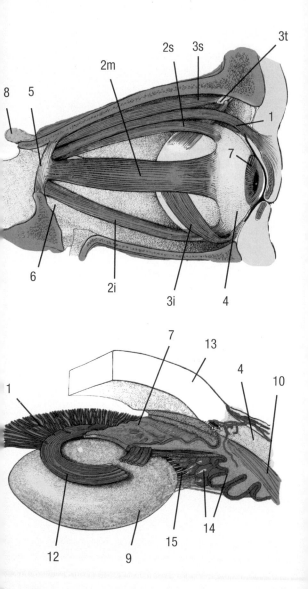

Muscles of the Eye
Coronal view

superficial T removed
EB contents removed - sclera intact
apex of the orbit - muscle bed intact

1. Levator Palpebrae Superioris m -
2. Recti m -
   - i = inferior / s = superior
   - L = lateral / m = medial
3. Oblique m
   - i = inferior / s = superior
4. trochlear N = CN IV
5. ciliary ganglion - sympathetic N travels via CN III
6. abducent N = CN VI
7. oculomotor N = CN III
8. trochlea
9. superior orbital notch
10. superior orbital fissure
11. optic N = CN II
12. lacrimal gld
13. CTR
14. sclera

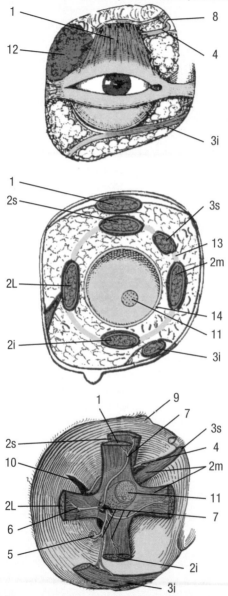

Movements of the EYE

All eye movements can be defined as rotations about the Fick's axes.

These are defined as lines drawn through the "centre" of the EB = 13.5mm behind the cornea in the ametropia - longer in myopia and shorter in hyperopia. This is the Centre of Rotation (C)

X - horizontal (transverse) axis from nasal to temporal,

Y - sagittal (in the eye) axis from the anterior to posterior poles - (note this is not the same as the sagittal plane of the body)

& Z - vertical axis from superior to inferior

The anterior pole is used as the ref point for all eye movements.

Single eye movements = DUCTIONS

Rotations around X - the horizontal axis - move the eye up or down - elevation & depression respectively

Rotations around Z - the vertical axis - move the eye towards the nasal or temporal sides - adduction & abduction respectively

Rotations around Y - the eye sagittal axis - rotate the eye inwards towards the nose or outwards towards to the temple - intorsion or extorsion and mainly these movements are to keep the eye focused on a particular object as the head tilts

Listing's plane (L) AKA the Equatorial plane is the frontal plane passing through the centre of rotation when the eye is looking straight ahead. Many movements take place in this plane. Changing of the EB gaze - fixation point creates a new equatorial plane from which all subsequent movements may be achieved, hence torsion as such is not needed but this does not hold for the eye maintaining fixation when the head moves. If the head moves but fixation is maintained then the eye must tort in the opposite direction. This fixation is maintained by the vestibulo-ocular reflex.

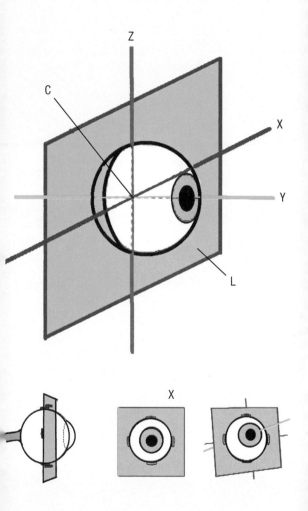

Z

C

X

Y

L

X

Movements of the EYE

Four of the EOMs are angulated in the eye socket when the eyes are in the primary position, so that on contraction they have primary & secondary movements, except LR & MR. These movements are described according to Fick's axes. Most of the muscles originate from the common tendinous ring (CTR) surrounding the ON & insert in a spiral around the anterior EB, further complicating their movements.

Muscle	Origin	Insertion	Primary Action	Secondary Action
MR	CTR +ON sheath	antero-medial EB	**Adduction**	None
LR	CTR greater wing of the Sphenoid	antero-lateral EB	**Abduction**	None
SR	CTR +ON sheath	superio-anterior EB	**Elevation**	Adduction, intorsion
IR	CTR	inferio-inferior EB	**Depression**	Adduction, extorsion
SO	lesser wing of the Sphenoid via the trochlea	superior/ posterior lateral EB	**Intorsion**	Depression, abduction
IO	medial Maxilla	inferior/ posterior lateral EB	**Extorsion**	Elevation, abduction

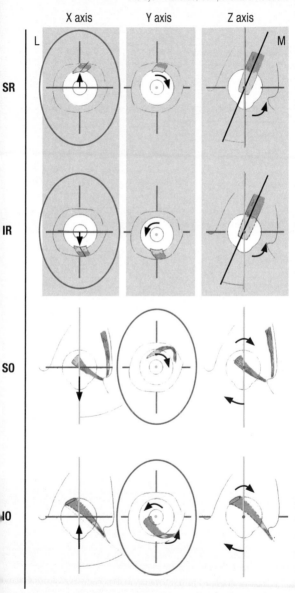

	X axis	Y axis	Z axis
SR	L		M
IR			
SO			
IO			

Movements of the EYE

Binocular movement - VERSIONS & VERGENCES

When both eyes are looking in the same direction, normal binocular movements require the cooperation of the yoke muscles. These are the primary agonist muscles pairs *1 from each eye* which ensure that the eyes are gazing in the same direction - **conjugate movements** or **VERSIONS,** as opposed to **disconjugate movements (VERGENCES)** where the eyes may be focusing on the same object but this requires their movements in opposite directions. The control of these coordinated movements - takes place in the cerebellum & brainstem, and from reflexes w/n the EOM. For each primary mover - **the agonist** there is also an equal suppression of its opposite muscle in the same eye. Many complex movements are actually a balance b/n all 6 of the EOMs.

Binocular

	Eye Movement	Term
1	Right	Dextroversion
2	Left	Levoversion
3	Up	Supravision sursumversion
4	Down	Infraversion deorsumversion
5	Up and right	Dextroelevation
6	Up and left	Levoelevation
7	Down and right	Dextrodepression
8	Down and left	Levodepression
9	Both eyes adduct	Convergance
not shown	Both eyes abduct	Divergence
	Both eyes extort	Excyclovergence
	Both eyes intort	Incyclovergence
	Rotation of 12-o'clock position to the right	Dextrocycloversion
	Rotation of 12-o'clock position to the left	Levocycloversion

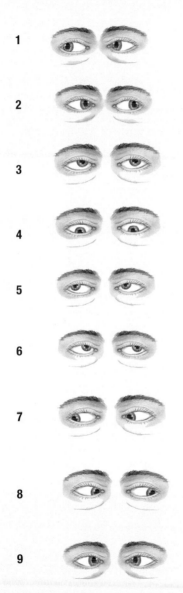

1

2

3

4

5

6

7

8

9

Optic Nerve – CN II
Chiasm

Schema

CN II is the special sense N which transmits afferent vision impulses to the brain. In binocular vision this involves a mixing and blending of the 2 slightly different images from each eye into one single vision with depth perception. The inner or nasally placed N fibres from each eye cross over to the contralateral optic tract and then to the visual cortex of the brain to facilitate this interpretation, while the outer or temporal fibres remain in the same tract – ipsilateral.

1   ON from one eye
2   loops in the crossing fibres
      a = anterior knee of Wilebrand
      p = posterior knee of Wilebrand
3   optic chiasm
4   optic tract
5   temporal fibres – from the lateral retina
      i = inferior
      s = superior
6   nasal fibres – from the medial retina
      i = inferior
      s = superior

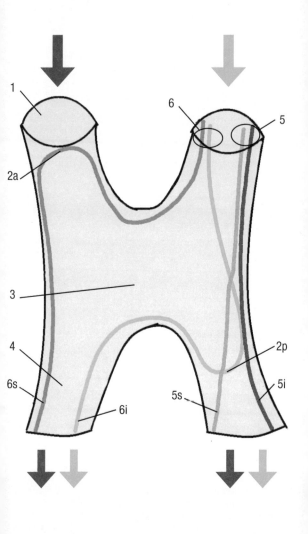

Optic Nerve – CN II
Blood Supply - arterial

Transverse - inf. Brain surface
Longitudinal - cut through the ON

The central retinal a & v travel with the ON, emerge at the OD & supply the upper layers of the retina - the lower 1/3 supplied by the choroid. There is no direct aa b/n these 2 supplies both are essential. The brain layers continue along CN II and merge with the layers of the sclera with the penetration of the ON into the EB.

1 central vessels of the retina a = artery v = vein
2 ophthalmic a
3 internal carotid
4 cerebral arteries a = anterior / m = middle /
   p = posterior branches
5 lateral striate a
6 optic radiation
7 visceral cortex
8 lateral geniculate body
9 optic tract
10 basilar a
11 anterior choroidal a
12 communicating artery a = anterior / p = posterior
13 superior hypophysial a
14 retina
15 choroid
16 sclera
17 short posterior ciliary arteries
18 Dura Mater
19 Arachnoid Mater
20 Pia Mater
21 subarachnoid space
22 plial plexus
23 central collateral a
24 circle of Zinn
25 lamina cribosa where CT of the sclera merges with the
    CNS CT

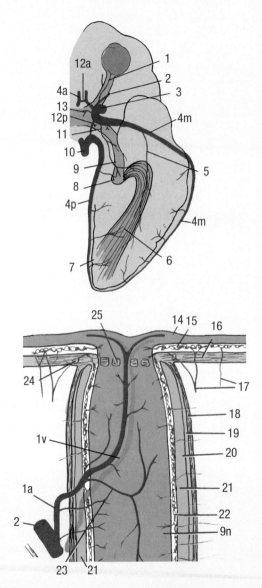

Optic Nerve – CN II
Intra-ocular part - the Optic Nerve Head

Longitudinal - cut through the ON

The optic N enters the EB as the OD - which is the physiological blind spot of the cye, bringing with It the central retinal BVs which supply the anterior layers of the retina. It is one of the 4 parts of the ON - and is ~ 1.5mm X 1.5mm in diameter. The Head as with the rest of the ON does not contain any N bodies only the axons from the neurons in the retina.

C = choriod

R = retina

S = sclera

N = Nasal side

T = Temporal side

1   retinal vessels a & v

2   optic pit - centre of the OD

3   astrocytes - in a nerve fascicle * b/n the N processes

4   cribiform plate - made up of CT

5   dura mater covering the ON

6   N fascicle containing ~1000 N fibres -all N axons from special sensory cells of the retina

7   CT septa b/n the fascicles derived from the pia mater & CT of the sclera

8   oligodendrocytes - supporting the fascicle

9   mantle surrounding the ON derived from all the meninges - mainly astrocytes

10 circle of Zinn

11 BM dividing the retina & choroid

12 Müller cells

13 OD - extent of the ON covered with astrocyte fibres

14 perivascular CT around the retinal BVs & continuous with cribiform plate

* astrocytes supporting each N process

T   N

12   13   14   1   2   3

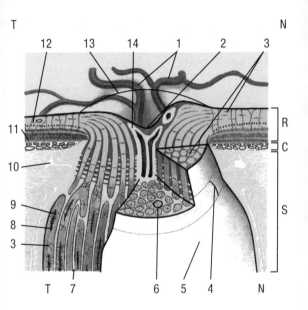

11

10

9

8

3

T   7   6   5   4   N

R

C

S

Orbital Fissure & Canal

Anterior view

The NS & the BS of the EB and its adnexae enter via the orbital fissure and canal.

1 supraorbital a
2 superior orbital fissure
3 supraorbital v
4 Lateral Rectus m
5 superior division of CN III
6 abducent N = CN VI
7 inferior division of CN III
8 inferior orbital fissure
9 infraorbital v
10 Inferior Rectus m
11 nasociliary N
12 Medial Rectus m
13 Superior Oblique m
14 ophthalmic a
15 Levator Palpabrae Superioris m
16 ON = CN II - in the orbital canal
17 trochlear N = CN IV
18 frontal N (br of CN V$_1$)
19 lacrimal N

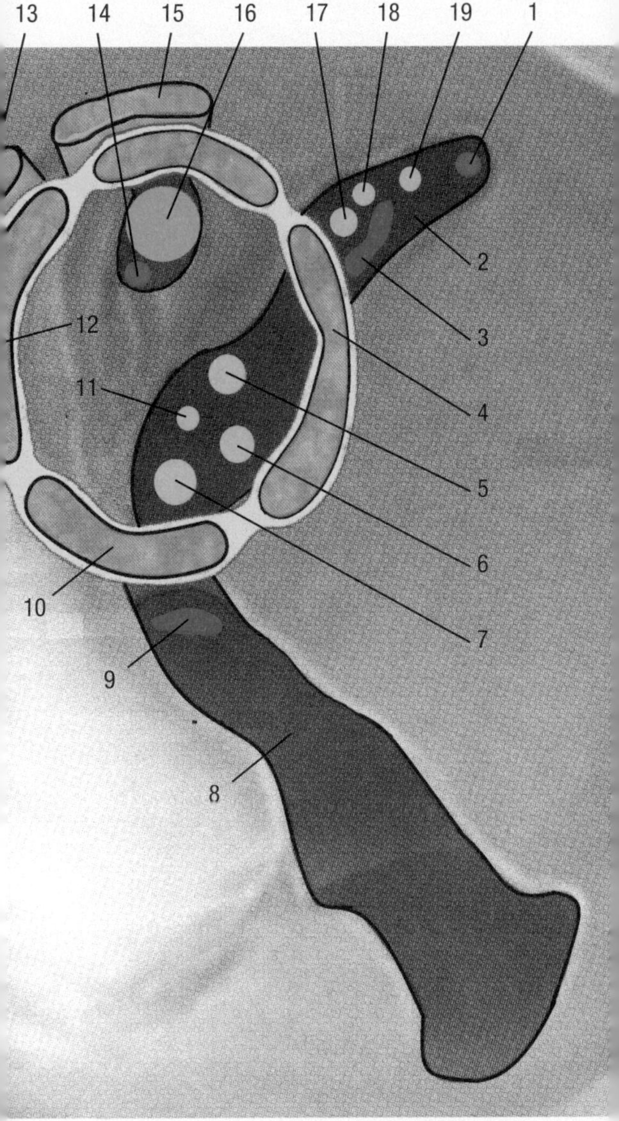
13
14
15
16
17
18
19
1
2
3
4
5
6
7
8
9
10
11
12

Orbital Fossa
Bones

Anterior - face on view of the bones of the orbital fossa
Lateral (L) & Medial (M) walls
Floor (F) & Roof (R) of the orbit

The bony orbit is composed of the meeting of several bones. The space is not a closed box as is the skull but there is limited space. The ON (CN II) passes through the apex of the fossa, while the other CNs pass through the orbital fissure.

Note the close proximity of the orbit to many sinuses in the skull, all of which may communicate with EB directly if perforated.

1 Sphenoid bone
   b = body
   g = greater wing
   L = lesser wing
   s = sinus
2 orbital fissure at the apex
   i = inferior
   s = superior
3 Frontal bone + its orbital plate makes up most of the roof of the orbit
   c = cribosa - or foramina from the frontal sinus
4 Optic canal (for ON)
5 superior orbital notch + foramen
6 Ethmoid bone
   f = ethmoidal foramina - from the ethmoid sinus
   s = ethmoid sinus
7 Lacrimal bone + duct (AKA Nasolacrimal canal)
8 Nasal bone
9 Inferior nasal concha
10 Maxilla + its orbital plate (p) - makes up most of the floor of the orbit
11 infra-orbital foramen
12 Palatine bone
13 Zygoma + its orbital plate - makes up most of the lateral wall of the orbit
14 pterygopalantine foramen / fossa
15 palatine canal
16 foramen rotundum

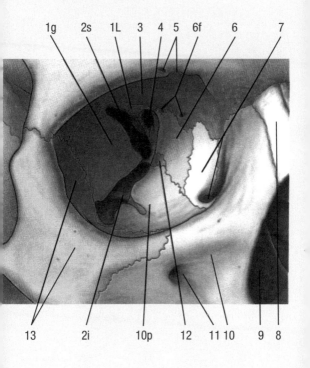

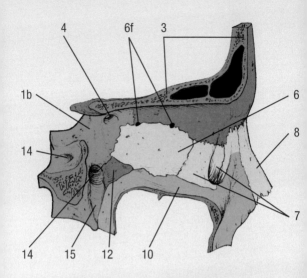

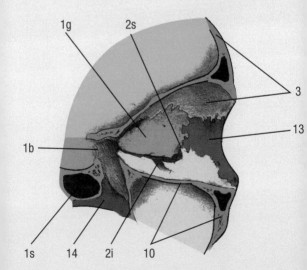

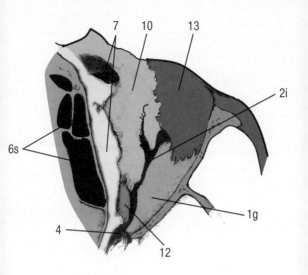

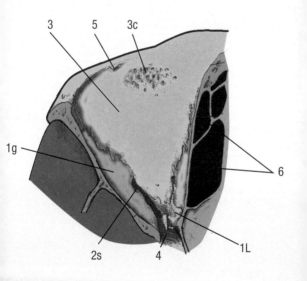

Orbit

Sinuses

Anterior / Lateral - looking onto the face with sinus projections from the front & the side
Coronal - slice through the apex of the skull to demonstrate bones sinuses
Superior - looking down on the ACF - top of the orbit

Because of the need to lighten the weight of the skull its bones have air pockets or sinuses, the orbit composed of many of these bones is surrounded by these thin-walled cavities. Confluence with surrounding structures including the nasal cavity make these areas susceptible to infections, and their thin walls make them vulnerable to trauma. In turn the orbit is also vulnerable to traumatic & inflammatory processes.

1. cranial vault at the ACF
2. ethmoid sinus / air cells
   - a = anterior
   - m = middle
   - p = posterior
   - i = infundibulum - communication with the maxillary sinuses
3. maxillary sinus
4. nasal cavity
5. bony palate = hard palate
6. inferior meatus (lacrimal duct opens at this level)
   - A = inferior concha
7. middle meatus (opening)
   - A = middle concha
8. superior meatus
   - A = superior concha
9. orbit = orbital fossa containing the EB & extra-ocular m
   - f = floor
10. frontal sinus
11. superior orbital plate - from Frontal bone
12. Sphenoid - greater wing (g) / lesser wing (L) sinus (s)
13. Crista galli -leading onto the nasal septum may be pneumatised
14. nasal septum & Vomer

■ Frontal bone components

■ Zygoma components

■ Maxilla components

■ Ethmoid bone components

■ Inferior nasal concha components

■ Vomer components

■ Sphenoid bone components

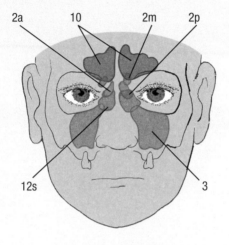

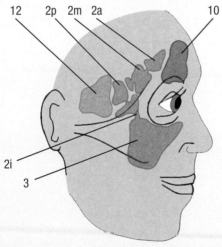

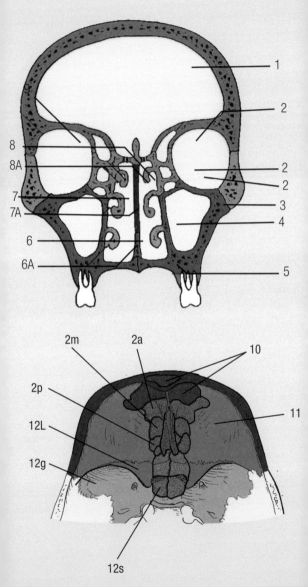

© A. L. Neill

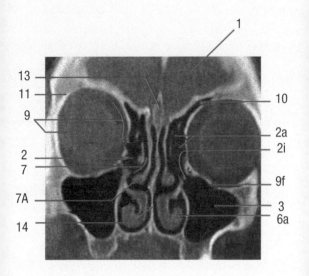

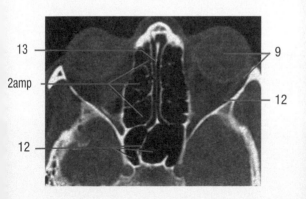

Pupil
Light Response

Schema

The pupil will respond along with the lens to focus when it is too near objects and too light - contracting in both cases for better VA.

The green lines show the efferent pathways to effect the response and the other lines indicate the afferent pathways of the retina.

1 ON
2 chiasm
3 optic tract
4 lateral geniculate body
5 superior brachium
6 pre-tectal nucleus
7 cerebral aqueduct
8 Edinger -Westphal nucleus
9 CN III - oculomotor N some brs. also carrying ANS fibres
10 ciliary ganglion
11 short ciliary Ns
12 posterior commissure

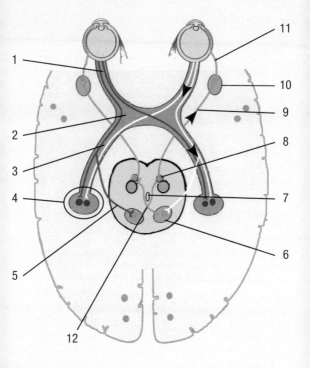

Pupil
Near Response / Accommodation Reflex

Schema

The pupil will respond along with the lens to focus when it is too near objects and too light - contracting in both cases for better VA.

The green lines show the efferent pathways to effect the response and the other lines indicate the afferent pathways of the retina.

1 ON
2 chiasm
3 optic tract
4 lateral geniculate body
5 fibres of the optic radiation
6 striate cortex of the occipital lobe
7 oculomotor nucelus - medial rectus subnucleus
8 Edinger - Westphal nucleus
9 fibres from the frontal eye fields
10 frontal eye fields
11 ciliary ganglion
12 short ciliary N
13 CN III - oculomotor N some branches carrying ANS fibres

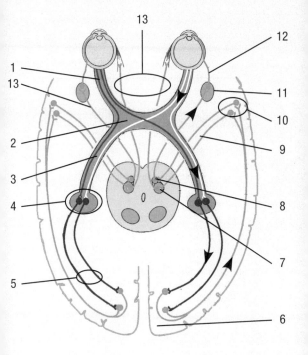

Retina

Schema

The retina has 9 distinct layers, seen clearly in sections and they are due to the highly organized nature of this specialized structure. These are in order from the retinal surface to the base:

ILM	internal limiting membrane
NFL	nuclear fibre layer
GCL	ganglion cell layer
IPL	inner plexiform layer
INL	inner nuclear layer
OPL	outer plexiform layer
ONL	outer nuclear layer
ELM	external limiting membrane
P	photoreceptors + pigmented epithelium intimately connected
L	direction of incident light

1	ganglion cell
2	amacrine cell
3	bipolar cell
4	horizontal cell
5	photoreceptive cell
6	specialized endings
	c = cones
	r = rods
7	RPE
8	Müller cells - supporting the specialist cells

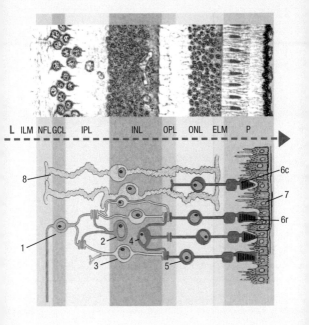

L   ILM NFL GCL   IPL   INL   OPL   ONL   ELM   P

8

1

2

4

3   5

6c

7

6r

Retina

development of neural layers and components

Müller cells removed for clarity. They span the full retinal thickness.

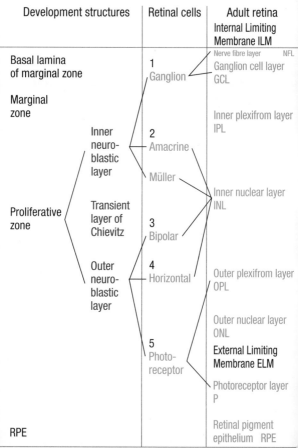

Development structures	Retinal cells	Adult retina
		Internal Limiting Membrane ILM
Basal lamina of marginal zone	1 Ganglion	Nerve fibre layer NFL
		Ganglion cell layer GCL
Marginal zone		Inner plexifrom layer IPL
Inner neuro-blastic layer	2 Amacrine	
	Müller	Inner nuclear layer INL
Proliferative zone	Transient layer of Chievitz	
	3 Bipolar	
Outer neuro-blastic layer	4 Horizontal	Outer plexifrom layer OPL
		Outer nuclear layer ONL
	5 Photo-receptor	External Limiting Membrane ELM
		Photoreceptor layer P
RPE		Retinal pigment epithelium RPE

222

© A. L. Neill

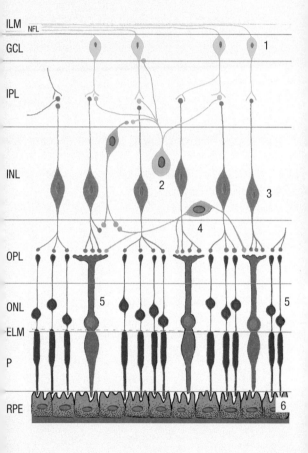

ILM
NFL
GCL   1

IPL

INL   2

                                                       3

OPL   4

ONL   5   5

ELM

P

RPE   6

Retina

Nerve distribution schema
View of the fundus of the retina showing neural pathways
Cross section of the ON just prior to the chiasm

The macula represents the area of central vision in the eye. It takes up about 1/20 of the area of the visual retina, but occupies 1/3 of the fibres in the OD & ON. The other areas the nasal & temporal regions occupy the other 2/3 equally. The N fibres do not cross but arc around to the OD and become more superficial closer to the macula, as the retina also thins. The fibres rotate in the ON and then in the chiasm further change the nasal fibres crossing to the contralateral side as they travel in the optic tract.

M	N fibres from the macula
N	N fibres from the nasal field (superior & inferior)
T	N fibres from the temporal field (superior & inferior)
OD =	optic disc (ONH)
ON =	CN II

1	blind spot
2	papillomacular fibre bundle
3	macula - macular axons

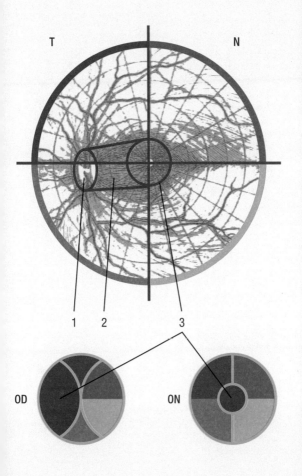

T   N

OD   ON

1   2   3

Retina

Communicating retinal cells
Amacrine cells

Amacrine cells reside in the IPL and facilitate communication w/n the retina facilitating additional connections b/n the bipolar & ganglion cells. Similar to the horizontal cells they facilitate communication across areas of the retina.

IPL   level of the inner plexiform layer of the retina

1   amarcrine cell
2   bipolar cell
3   ganglion cell
4   amarcrine – bipolar axon-axon contact
5   amarcrine – ganglion axon-soma contact
6   bipolar ganglion axon-soma contact
7   dyad contact – 3 cells interconnecting

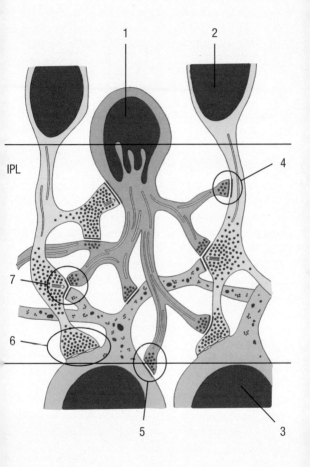

IPL

Retina

Communicating retinal cells
Bipolar & Horizontal cells

There are a number of different types of cellular communication in the retina. Many via bipolar cells - cells with one axon and one dendrite communicate with only one rod or cone cell and travel to specific region in the lateral geniculate body. These single communicating cone bipolar cells are concentrated in the macular and foveal regions to allow for sharp precise visual signals. Horizontal cells have long flat processes which traverse over many cells and communicate with them all and these cells are involved in the assimilation of visual signals from several cells.

IPL level of the inner plexiform layer of the retina

1 rod bipolar cells may communicate with several rod cells

2 midget bipolar cells - concentrate on only one cone cell in the fovea - for sharp specific visual detail

3 horizontal cells - long branches with many processes for visual integration b/n rods & cones

4 flat bipolar cells - over several cones in the outer regions - subgroups labelled according to the region in the lat. geniculate body to which they correspond

5 cone cells
> p = pedicles which may have input from several ganglion cells

6 rod cells
> s = sphericles which have fewer ganglion contacts than cone cells

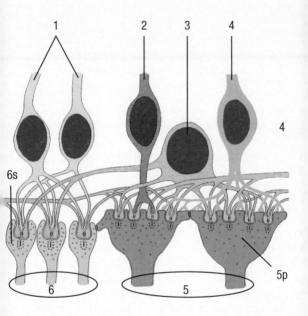

Retina

Supportive retinal cells
Müller cells

Müller cells have many features of glia. Long columnar cells they extend from the inner retinal surface to beyond the ELM. Their nuclei are found at the level of the INL.

A = apical region – long & thin, devoid of organelles

B = basal region – shorter wider enclosing N cell processes – dendrites and axons w/n their cytoplasm

ELM = level of the external limiting membrane

1   terminal villous process of the cell

2   tight junctional complexes with the adjacent rod & cone cells

3   mitochondria – small & round in the apex, long & plentiful in the base

4   GA

5   process to enclose the axons &/or dendrites of adjacent N cells

6   cytoplasmic filaments – much denser in the basal regions

7   BM

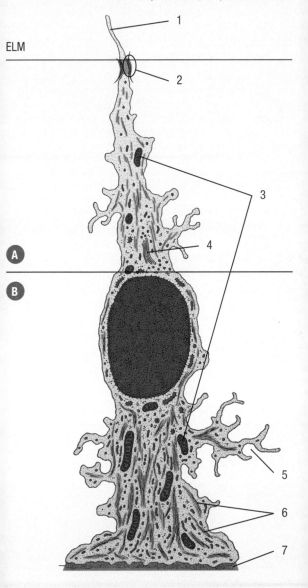

ELM

A

B

1

2

3

4

5

6

7

Retina

Supportive retinal cells
Retinal Pigmented Epithelium (RPE)

The RPE is a highly pigmented layer of modified cuboidal epithelial cells which cover & nourish the specialized endings of the rod & cone cells of the retina, preventing them from being exposed to stray light in the retina. The melanin pigment absorbs stray light in the globe, preventing reflections & dispersed light from interfering with the retinal image. This epithelium forms the outer layer of the retina and lies on Bruch's membrane. It is supplied by the choroidal BVs.

1. microvilli – much longer than the usual mv which wrap themselves around the endings of the rods & cones
2. melanin granules in the apical region & in mv
3. RER – much less plentiful than the SER and clear vesicles in the cell
4. laminated bodies – pre-melanin granules, found in the base of the cell
5. BM – part of Bruch's membrane
6. GA
7. mitochondria

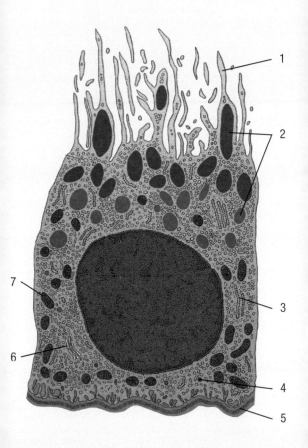

1

2

2

3

7

6

4

5

Retina

Specialized sensory cells -
Cones (C)
Rods (R)

The retina consists of a number of specialist cells which together are responsible for the initial input to form visual perception. The special sensory cells are the CONES (C) and the RODS (R), so named because of the shape of their outer apical segments. Rs are more sensitive to movement and respond to dim light more than Cs which perceive colour & shape better and this is the reason they are concentrated in the region of the fovea and its centre foveola, whereas Rs are found more in the periphery of the retina " the corner of the eye". These cells have different visual pigments (R= rhodopsin / C = iodopsin) but the excitation of the apical end in either, initiates VP.

1 outer apical segment consists of parallel membranous lamellae
    R longer than C
    C wider then R
    lamellae R encapsulated / C not encapsulated

2 modified cilial stalk connecting segments - R>C

3 inner segment
    junction b/n 3 & 4 is a junctional complex with the Müller cells site of the ELM

4 outer fibre - R>C

5 cell body - C>R

6 inner fibre - R>C

7 rod spherule / cone pedicel
    site of the junction with the horizontal cells &/or bipolar cells - C>R

8 synaptic vesicles C>R

9 synaptic ribbons - vesicles surrounding the deeply inserted N fibrils from the bipolar cells in the retina

10 microtubules

11 GA & ribosomes C>R

12 mito C>R

13 inserted process of the horizontal cells - 3 in the C, 1 in R

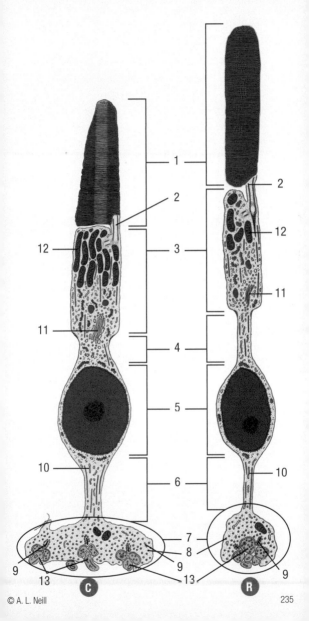

© A. L. Neill

Tear Film (TF)
Structure

The TF has 3 layers: the Meibomian glands - the thin surface lipid layer; the lacrimal glands - the bulk of the film - the aqueous layer (80-90%) & the goblet cells of the glands of the EL - the thin mucoid layer which is adherent to the corneal surface epithelium.

With drying the upper & lower layers mix & cause the TF breakdown exposing the cornea & sclera.

Functions : oxygen supply of the surface corneal epithelium; smooth passage of the upper EL across the cornea & the even refractive surface of the cornea. The TF is re-established with every blink - breaks down b/n 15-40 sec, due to the lacrimal pump mechanism, which also allows for the continual drainage of the tear film.

Tear production ↓ by 60% after 65yo which may or may not cause dry eyes but renders the person more susceptible to this disease; exacerbated by air conditioners, blinking disorders, windy weather conditions, pollution, medications & the wearing of CLs.

1 lipid layer - prevents excessive evaporation
2 aqueous layer - thickest portion provides and even refractile surface
3 mucoid / aqueous transition
   s = mucoid strands usually unnoticeable - thicker & ropier in dry eye syndrome
4 microvilli
5 surface corneal epithelium - flattened wing cells are tightly bound to prevent any leakage of the tear into the corneal T - which would disrupt the stroma and render the cornea cloudy

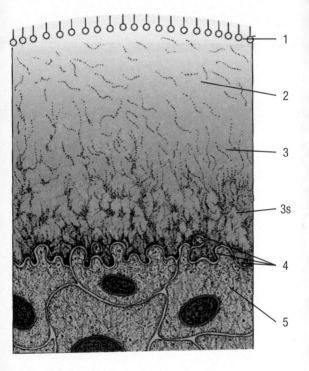

1

2

3

3s

4

5

Vitreous Body

Schema

LP

HP

The VB is a gel made up of ~ 99% water, hyaluronic acid & collagen fibres. It lies behind the lens fills most of the posterior chamber of the eye – the vitreous chamber. The strongest attachment is b/n the vitreous base and the ora serrata. The CB zonules are intertwined with the collagen fibres of the VB. The VB only attaches to BM material. The VB if removed is not replaced or repaired by the body but maybe replaced with water, often leading to cataracts & floaters.

1. entrance of the ON = ONH
2. hyaloid channel AKA retrolental canal – runs in an S-shape along the length of the EB in the wake of the embryonic hyaloid BV system – long unbranched collagen strands course around this area and form the attachments to the structures at the back of the EB & the back of the lens
3. intermediate zone – collagen fibres run along the length of the EB
4. vitreous cortex – outer zone – hyaloid collagen fibres are at right angles to the CB and retinal surface ~100µm note the collagen of the VB intertwines with the zonules of the CB
5. ora serrata - non visual 1/3 of the retina
6. crystalline lens
7. CB
8. a = ant. chamber, p = post. chamber
9. cornea
10. Berger's space – the internal space w/n the ring of the VB attachment to the back of the lens – it ↑ with age as the attachments of the VB decrease – rather than a true hole it is a fluid / water filled space devoid of the collagen fibres of the VB
11. collagen fibres in the outer zone coming out from the BM of the RPE
12. sclera
13. space b/n retina & VB replaced with fluid

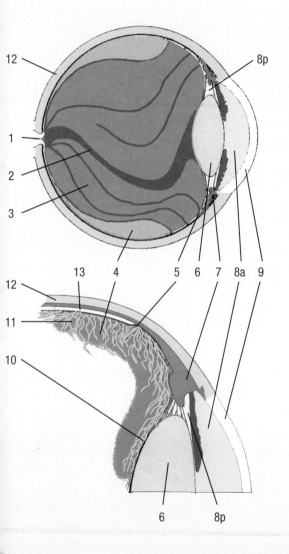

Asthenopia symptoms and possible aetiologies

Symptoms indicating urgency

Diplopia	Myasthenia gravis
	Thyroid disorders
	DM
	Third nerve palsy from any cause
Flashes of light	Retinal detachment
Sudden loss of vision	Macular degeneration
	Retinal artery occlusion
	Retinal detachment
	Retinal vein occlusion
	Retrobulbar neuritis
Transient	Carotid artery disease
	Migraine
	Papilloedema
	Severe hypertension
Pain in the eye	Chemical burn
	Flash burn to cornea
	Keratitis
	Glaucoma
	Iritis
	Temporal arteritis
	Retrobulbar neuritis
Ptosis	Third nerve palsy
	DM
	Myasthenia gravis
Trauma	Blow-out fracture of orbit
	Hyphaema

Symptoms requiring prompt attention

Blurred vision in the elderly	Macular degeneration Cataracts Ischemic optic neuropathy
Discharge and matting of lids in morning	Conjunctivitis
Enlarging nodule on lid	Basal cell carcinoma
Foreign body sensation	Corneal FB Corneal abrasion Herpes simplex keratitis
Halos around lights	Angle-closure glaucoma Cataracts
Persistent tearing in one eye	Dacryocystis Blocked tear duct Entropion, ectropion Trichiasis Chalazion Bell's palsy
Red eye	Any external disease of eye
Swelling of lids	Bilateral blepharoconjunctivitis Acute allergies Thyroid disease

Asthenopia symptoms and possible aetiologies *(continued)*

Significant symptoms that should be seen as soon as possible

Blurred distance vision in adult	DM
	Cataract
	Macular oedema
Eruption on skin	Atopic allergy
	Seborrhea
	Herpes zoster
	Drug reaction
Gritty feeling	Dry eye syndrome from any cause
	Conjunctivitis
	Ocular irritation - dust, wind, ultraviolet lights
Headaches	Often tension
	Hypertension
	Brain tumor
	Migraine, cluster headaches, etc.
Pain behind eye	Sinus disease
	Thyroid disorders
	Orbital tumor (rare)
	Aneurysm of the carotid artery (rare)
Spots before eye	Retinal tear
	Vitreous detachment

Cataract Surgery

1 - EB with opaque cataract
2 - Lifting of the cornea & opening of lens bag
3 - Exposure of the lens
4 - Pressure on the EB - pushes out the lens
5 - Clearing out of the lens bag
6 - Attachment of the new lens

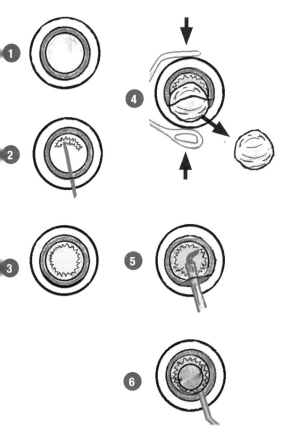

Cataract
Age-related

A - ant. & lat. views of coronary cataract
B - lat. view nuclear sclerotic cataract
C - lat. view cuneiform cataract (wedge-shaped)
D - lat. view posterior subcapsular cataract
E - lat. view Morgagnian cataract

A cataract is any opacity of the crystalline lens in the eye. It is thought to be due to ↑ protein precipitants in the lens with age. It is the commonest form of blindness in the elderly, affecting all forms of VA. Most forms of age-related cataracts are slow to progress & do not interfere in the early stages with VA.

A **mature** cataract indicates opacity throughout the lens, an **immature** cataract has some lucent areas & the **hypermature** cataract has liquefied cortical proteins which leak out of the lens capsule, causing it to wrinkle & develop further more severe opacities. If the lens is so shrunken that it floats about in the capsule it is a **Morgagnian** cataract (end-stage).

Primary cataracts are not related to other conditions in the body. Most age-related cataracts are primary.

1   pupil showing lens in the aperture
2   iris
3   capsule
       a = anterior wall
       p = posterior wall
4   cortex
5   nucleus
       o = opacified
       s = hardened / sclerosed
6   cortical spokes
7   peripheral opacities
       club endings - thicken rather than spread around the cortex
       spicule endings - spreading over more of the circumference
8   posterior subcapsular opacities (usually protein deposits)
L   direction of incident light

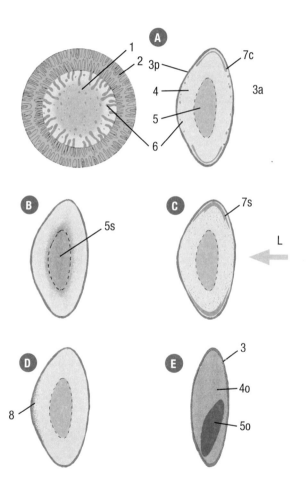

Cataract
Grading System for Age-related cataracts

The severity of the cataract can be determined by an examination of 3 factors found in most cataracts: nuclear sclerosis - or hardening shown in cross-section, corneal spoking -which are protein opacities starting at the lens's periphery spreading into the centre & around the circumference & the amount of protein deposits on the posterior lens &/or capsular surface. The opacities are seen in retroillumination.

The Tx for all forms of cataract is the removal of the lens & replacement with an artificial lens. Hence the VL must be severe enough to warrant this intervention, although there is no means to reverse or prevent cataract formation at this stage.

Common signs & symptoms include:

- Binocular & monocular diplopia, ± coloured halos

- Blurred vision which cannot be corrected with glasses for both near & far distance

- Poor dark adaptation & hypersensitivity to glare

- Reduced contrast & colour differentials

Lens removal can be done in a number of ways. Removal via the anterior or posterior capsule or from phakoemulsification (emulsifying the lens and then "sucking" it out anteriorly) being the commonest currently.

Most forms try to preserve at least part of the lens capsule so that the intraocular lens can be held in place. Preservation of the posterior wall of the lens capsule, can lead to "after cataract"- opacities which develop in the posterior capsule wall from remnants of the lens or direct protein deposits.

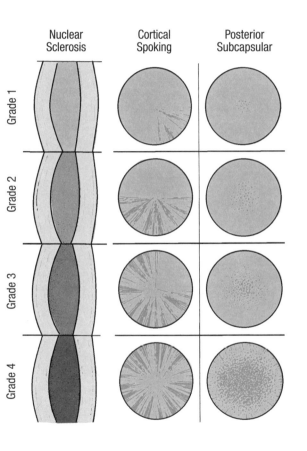

	Nuclear Sclerosis	Cortical Spoking	Posterior Subcapsular
Grade 1			
Grade 2			
Grade 3			
Grade 4			

Cataract
Secondary cataracts &
Primary congenital cataracts

A congenital cataract - zonular type
B contusional cataract - develops after trauma, FB & other blunt trauma
C contusional cataract with capsular perforation
D cataract assoc with intraocular disease ↑ IOP , uveitis etc.
E cataract assoc. with systemic disease e.g. DM
F "after cataract" development of post. capsular opacities

Congenital cataracts develop in the nucleus rather than the cortex.

Secondary cataract formation is associated with medications e.g. long term steroid use; other intraocular diseases e.g. glaucoma, uveitis; systemic diseases e.g. DM; trauma, including blunt trauma & FBs; toxins, e.g. workplace toxins and non-use of safety goggles; ↑ IOP & ↑ UV exposure.

These cataracts progress much faster and are more severe, interfering with the VA even in their early stages.

1 capsule
a = anterior wall
i = iris pigment ± remnants
o = opacities in posterior wall
p = posterior capsular wall
w = wrinkly capsule because of dissolved & leached out proteins
2 cortex
3 nucleus
o = opacified
4 stellate cataract
5 nuclear cataract
6 anterior subcapsular cataract
7 dot opacities
8 artificial lens
L direction of incident light

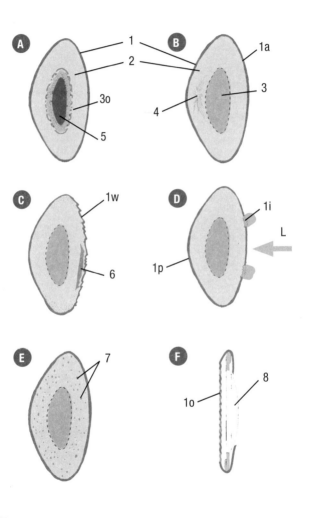

Conjunctivitis

The table indicates the incidence(%) & severity of symptoms (0-+++++)-in the various forms of conjunctivitis. Note often there is a mixed pathology in this disease, so the actual percentages may vary because of this,& individual variation. Most forms are highly contagious & have a high incidence in childhood. Cleanliness, isolation of cases & speedy treatment are recommended as the longer the duration of the disease the higher the chances of some residual loss of VA

	Allergic	Bacterial	Hyperbacterial / Acute	Viral
1	10% +	50% ++	60% +++	10% ++
2	30% +++	80% +++	100% ++++	80% +++
3	50% ++++	30% +	80% ++	60% +++++
4	30% +++++	50% ++++	-	10% ++
5	-	60% +++++	100% +++++	20% ++
6	100% ++++	30% ++	20% ++++	30% ++++
7	50% +++++	100% +++	100% +++++	60% +++
8	100% +++++	10% ++	20% ++	10% +++
9	-	50% ++	50% +++++	50% ++
10	10% ++	50% ++++	100% +++++	50% ++

1 follicles -swollen nodules under the EL
2 erythema - conjunctival injection near the limbus
3 watery discharge
4 mucoid discharge
5 purulent discharge with crusting on the eyelashes
6 swelling / itching
7 erythema of the bulbar conjunctiva
8 FB sensation -
9 photophobia / pain on EB movement
10 blurred vision clearing on blinking

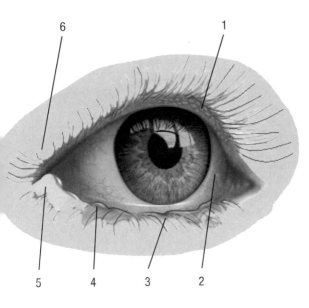

Contact Lenses (CL)

A - schema insertion of CL
B - comparison b/n HCLs & SCLS with movement of the EB
C - comparison b/n HCLs & SCLs with FBs

Approximately 20% of the population is myopic and presbyopia increases with age. Hence the number of people needing optical aids such as CL is increasing. CLs come in several forms but the main ones are soft (SCL) & hard (HCL).

HCLs cover only the central portion of the cornea, have a tight fit & cause local oedema in the region. They are easily dislodged, do not facilitate EL movement, but they are highly accurate & reproducible.

Both are inserted in a similar manner the ELs must be fully separated & the CL on a finger(s) is placed on the cornea.

SCLs have the following advantages over HCLs :
- they cause less corneal damage & cover the entire cornea preventing the entrance of FBs
- they are more comfortable & can be worn for longer periods
- they rarely dislodge so there are fewer losses & they are more suitable for sport
- they have less glare & photophobic symptoms

For most conditions SCLs are preferred, although they have some disadvantages:
- they cannot correct severe astigmatism;
- variable vision is experienced with eye movement
- not as precise or durable as HCLs
- lead to the formation of protein deposits on the cornea with excessive use
- cannot be modified or reproduced as accurately as the HCLs
- harder to disinfect & keep clean

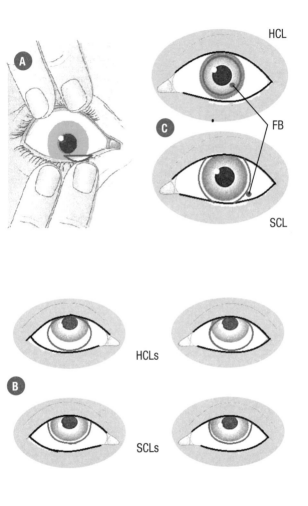

HCL

C

FB

SCL

HCLs

B

SCLs

Diagnostic fields of gaze & Muscle movements

A Description of muscle movements in a single eye
B Muscles responsible for movements from the primary gaze
C Muscles responsible for movement from positions of
abduction & adduction

There are 9 positions of gaze moving from the primary gaze position, which are used to test the presence of any EOM weakness, diplopia or other visual disturbances. The movements of the EOMs are described as either direct or torsional (curved) movements, using the anterior pole - or primary gaze as a reference.

Most EOMs move the EB in at least 2 directions: a direct & torsional movement, but the resultant eye movement also varies if the initial position is changed.

Note the description of eye movements changes when considering the eyes as a pair rather than the eye as a single entity.

Note the yoke muscle pairs.

L = Lateral / M = Medial

1   adduction
2   abduction
3   elevation / supraduction
4   depression / infraduction
5   intorsion / incycloduction
6   extortion / excycloduction

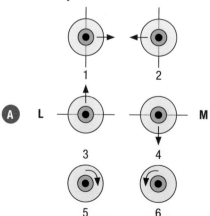

© A. L. Neill

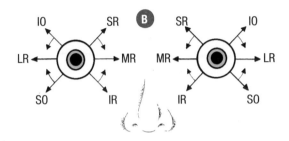

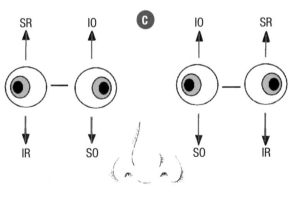

Drusen

Histology
HP H&E

Drusen are small colloidal globules w/n the Bruch's membrane b/n the mebrane & RPE of the retina. They contain lipids & proteins derived from the BS as well as trace elements - in particular Zn, which may be derived from the RPE. They increase with age, present in nearly all retinas > 40yo, but their sudden ↑ in numbers & size is an indicator of AMD if not a cause of it by disassociating the retina from its BS.

The small hard Druse shown here may become a large soft Druse by coalescing with other Drusen or expanding with time, resulting in retinal cell death.

1 **ONL**
2 **layer of rods & cones intimately related to ...**
3 **RPE**
4 **Bruch's membrane**
5 **choriocapillaris = capillary network of the choroid**
6 **choroid**
7 **hard druse**

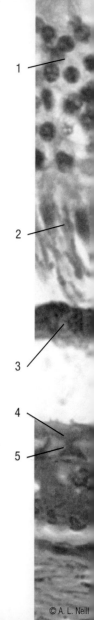

© A. L. Neill

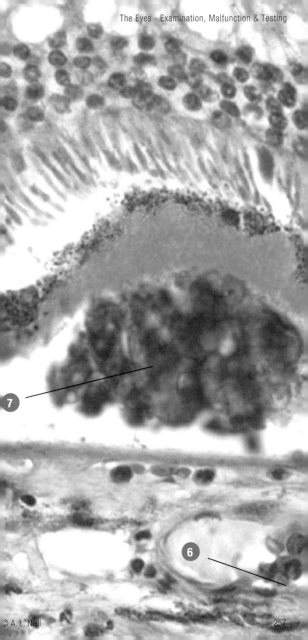

Eyedrop installation

Schema -

A instillation - tilt the head back

B avoiding the cornea - point to the lower EL cavity

C closure of the ELs - allowing for the effective spread

D reducing drainage - pressure on the medial canthus prevents drainage through the LA

Eyedrops are commonly prescribed & often poorly administered. The following show the method to produce the best results.

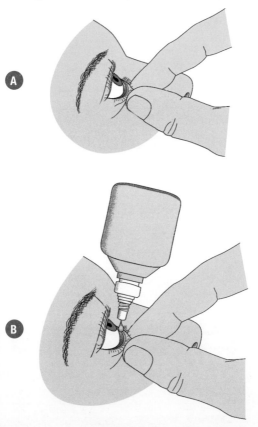

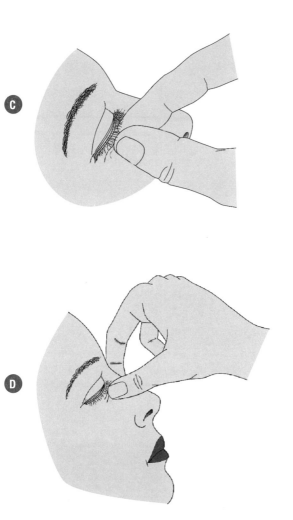

Glaucoma

A - mechanism of primary glaucoma (chronic)
B - mechanism of secondary glaucoma (chronic)

Glaucoma is a disease caused by ↑ IOP, hence ↓ BS of the retina, ↑ OD cupping, resulting in permanent VL. AH drainage is blocked due to the ↓ in the angle of the cornea & the iris = **ant. chamber angle (ACA)**.

Type	Cause	Symptoms	Comments
Primary open-angle	Gradual blockage of drainage channel; pressure builds slowly	Gradual loss of side vision; affects side vision first	Progresses very slowly and is a lifelong condition; considered the 'thief in the night'
Primary angle-closure	Total blockage of drainage channel; sudden increase in pressure	Nausea, blurred vision, severe pain. halos around lights	A medical emergency as permanent blindness occurs rapidly without immediate treatment
Secondary	Injury, infection, tumors, drugs, or inflammation, which causes scar tissue growth, blocking the drainage channel	Gradual loss of side vision; affects side vision first	May progress slowly; similar to chronic open-angle glaucoma
Congenital (infantile)	Fluid drainage system abnormal at birth	Light sensitivity, excessive tearing, enlarged eyes. cloudy cornea	Must be treated soon after birth if vision is to be saved

1. chambers of the eye
   a = anterior chamber
   p = posterior chamber
2. iris
   b = iris bombè (bowed up due to adhesions from previous If processes as in iritis / uveitis)
   r = raised iris due to ↑ IOP the lower the angle b/n the iris and the cornea the more likely there is to be closure & reduced drainage of the AH
   i = ACA <10° - closure present
   ii = ACA <30° - closure possible
   iii = ACA 30-45° closure improbable
3. cornea / limbus
4. canal of Schlemm
5. lens
6. CB
7. VB

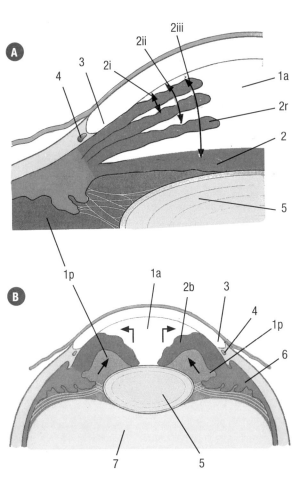

Macular Degeneration (MD)

Schema WET MD AKA Exudative MD

MD is a group of degenerative diseases of the retina that cause progressive, painless loss of central vision, due to the build up of substances b/n the special sensory vision cells & their BS - which comes from the RPE. If the build up of deposits is slow in & around the membrane it is DRY MD. These particles - Drusen prevent the diffusion of nutrients to these very sensitive cells, and patches of the RPE die leaving yellow gaps in the retina around the macular region.

The choroid BVs driven by anoxia & the IR may develop new BVs, leaky disorganized capillaries by neovascularization at any time. These capillaries break through the membranes & push through to the retina weeping protein exudates throughout the deep retinal layers aggressively disrupting the photosensitive layer causing severe & sudden VL. This is WET MD.

1. retinal special sensory cells
   - c = cone cells
   - r = rod cells
2. RPE
   - d = dead / dying RPE
3. Bruch's membrane
4. choriocapillaris = capillaries in the choroid
   - n = new BVs sprouting from a choroid vessel - neovascularization
   - p = thin-walled disorganised new capillary beds these can be found beneath the RPE, above the RPE & onto the retinal surface
5. Drusen
6. exudates - protein fluid leaking from the new BVs
7. Hgs from the weak capillaries - may be seen on the retinal surface - push and distort the orientation of the rods & cones
8. developing separation of layers in the retina & b/n the rods & cones from BV leakage

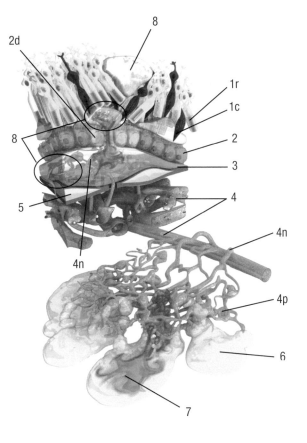

Optic Cupping / OD pallor

Schema

A - EB with ↑ OP

B - moderate cupping - ~ 0.5

C - severe cupping >0.9

D - 6 images showing progressive cupping and OD pallor from normal D_1 to end-stage D_6

The normal "cup " is the slight depression with a smooth rim at the site of the emergence of the ON (ONH). There is a large variation in the extent of this in the normal eye, so a better measure is the cup to disc ratio which is about 0.5, and if this ratio progresses associated with OD pallor, it is pathognomonic of glaucoma.

With the deepening and elongation of the "cup" and "sharpening of its rim, the BVs are crushed as they are pressed onto the rim depriving the retinal cells - the ganglion cells in particular of their BS. Progressively the OD becomes paler with irreversible VL.

1   anterior chamber
2   developing cup
3   ON
4   rim of the cup -beginning on the temporal side - but extending throughout

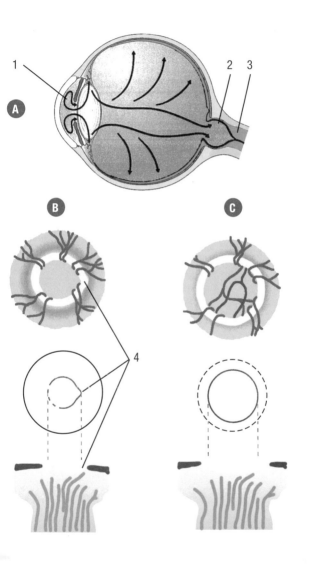

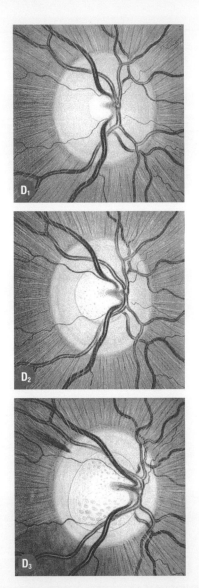

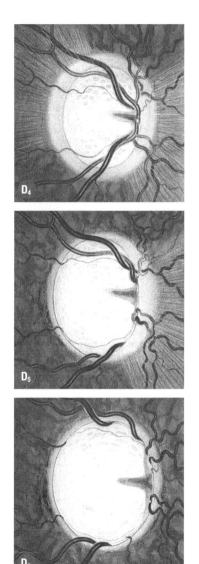

The Red Eye

Sign / Symptom	Conjunctivitis		
	Allergic	**Bacterial**	**Viral**
Conjunctiva	Mild BV dilatation	Diffuse BV dilatation	
Cornea	NAD		
Discharge	Watery	Purulent	Mucoid
IOP	NAD		
Pain	Severe itching	Itching mild pain	Itching mild pain
Pupil	NAD		
Vision	NAD		

Episcleritis	Glaucoma Acute angle	Subconjunctival Haemorrhage	Uveitis / Iritis
Patchy Hgs	BV dilatation at the Limbus	Patchy Hgs	BV dilatation at the Limbus
NAD	Shallow angle - Maybe cloudy	NAD	Deposits on cornea inner surface
Nil			
NAD	↑	NAD	↑ or ↓
Moderate	Severe	Nil	Severe
NAD	Mid-dilated	NAD	Constricted
NAD	↓ - Halos Loss of PV	NAD	Clouding of vision

Pupils - Examination

Shape & Size

Pupils are equal and circular b/n 3-5mm in diameter in normal room light.

DIFFERENT SIZES
Anisocoria - see Adie's pupil

THE CONTRACTED PUPIL
Drug-induced
Horner's syndrome (sympathetic paralysis) - contracted pupil more obvious in dim light + ptosis

Iritis - ± ciliary flush ± KPs ± irregular shape ± iris / lens adherence (post. synechiae)

THE DILATED PUPIL - (malfunction of the iris sphincter)
Adie's pupil - pupil responds to near focus > to light - may always appear as larger than the normal pupil

Drug induced
Glaucoma- ↑ IOP, ± distorted shape - oval

Third Nerve Palsy - pupil also down & out, poorly reactive + ptosis - Ix intracranial lesions

Trauma -+ associated ly to the surrounding Ts

Tests

Swinging Flashlight Test - the Direct & Consensual Light Reflexes

1   a light is shone directly into the defective eye (D) in a dimly lit room
2   both eyes normal (N) & defective (D) contract to a minimum size (over compensation) 2mm
3   both eyes then adjust to the light the intermediate size (escape) 3mm
4   the light is then moved quickly to the N eye - 2mm direct & consensual constriction BUT
5   MOVED BACK TO D - paradoxical dilatation OCCURS IN BOTH EYES due to slowing in D of afferent signal 4mm

No reaction to light but accommodates - Argyll -Robertson pupil
No reaction to direct light but consensual reaction intact - Marcus Gunn pupil - ON ± retinal disease
No reaction to light - local injury /effects - iris sphincter paralysis ± CN III palsy

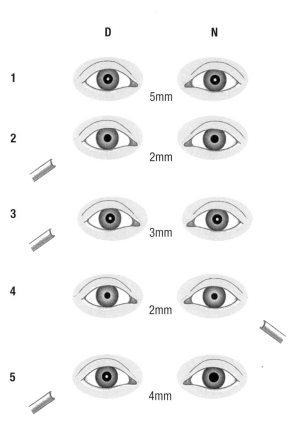

D   N

1   5mm

2   2mm

3   3mm

4   2mm

5   4mm

Refractive Errors (RE)

REs occur when one or both of the 2 major refractive components (the cornea or lens) do not align with the shape of the EB, so that the incident light cannot be focused to a sharp point on the back of the retina. The patient will report inability to focus, diplopia or other focus changes. Negative lenses (concave) will correct the myope - large pupil - with focus before the fovea & positive lenses (convex) will correct the hyperope - small pupil - with a focus longer than the EB.

However irregularities of the cornea &/or lens will result in irregular - or dispersed focus which is harder to correct. Cylindrical lenses may need to be inserted in various planes of the corrective lens.

Using the rectinoscope irregularities can be detected in the pupillary reflex which indicate the type & extent of RE. The duller & more dispersed the reflex the more severe the RE.

1 normal eye shows a strong bright defined reflex which follows the retinoscope in all directions

2 hyperope - "with" movement with the light

3 myope - "against" movement - moving in the opposite direction from the light

4 astigmatism & other irregularities* - reflex does not follow the retinoscope predictably & is irregular

5 neutralization point - when there is no movement & the pupil is filled with a red glow

* other conditions which demonstrate RE include: cataracts, corneal scarring, dirty or poorly fitting CL, corneal warping including keratoconus & lens subluxation

1

2

3

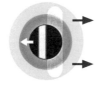

4

5

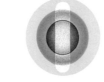

Reflexes
Blink & Corneal reflexes

Schema

The EL is the protective covering of the EB. Hence anything threatening or appearing to threaten the EB will cause an immediate protective response - blinking.

Tapping of the glabella; sudden shining of bright light and touching of the cornea will all illicit a reflex blinking, as well as any strong emotional stimulus. There may also be pupillary changes.

1. stimuli for the reflex - bright light / corneal touch / tapping of glabella
2. afferent input to trigger the reflex from ON & ophthalmic N (CN V$_1$)
3. afferent input from the higher emotional centres
4. motor nucleus of CN VII
   f = fibres of CN VII
5. sensory nucleus of CN V
6. midbrain visual reflex centre
7. Orbicularis Oculi m - responsible for tight reflex blinking (innervation CN VII)

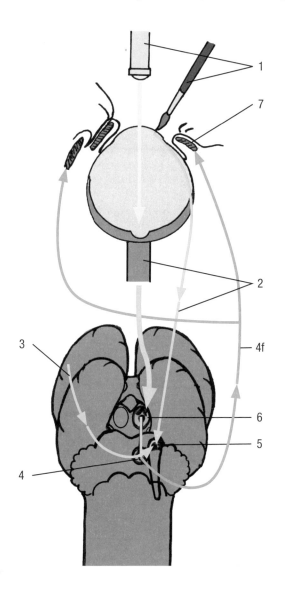

Retinopathy
Retinal Detachment

A retinal tear - anterior fundal view
B retinal detachment - sagittal view

The retina is a series of cellular & fibrous layers ending in the embedding of the ends of the special sensory cells (rods & cones) in the processes of the RPE, which is supplied by nutrients & oxygen diffusing from the choroid BVs. Pressure from the VB pulling on the retina to which it is loosely attached can tear the retina apart separating it from the RPE layer - the rod & cone BS. This tugging of the retinal layers can present as a series of flashes & lines, or as a sudden increase in the number & size of floaters. Most retinal tears occur in the periphery sparing the macula (to which the VB is not attached) hence the resulting VL may not be noticed by the patient until the tear has become more extensive, and permanent. Without being re-fixed to the base the vitreous humour can move in behind the lifted retinal layers & prevent their re-attachment. This will result in permanent VL & local weakness of the retinal layers, allowing for further separation.

1 retinal neural layer
2 RPE - base retinal layer (often thought of as part of the choroid)
3 choroid
4 sclera
5 OD
6 fundus
7 supf. retinal layers
    d = detachment of the top layers
    t = retinal tear
8 ON

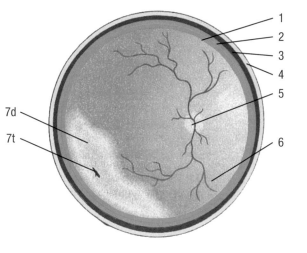

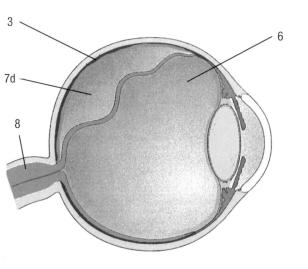

Blunt Trauma
Blow-out fracture

Anterior view - CT scan

Sagittal view – schema

A blow-out fracture is caused by blunt trauma onto the bony orbit (eg. ball hitting the eye). The orbital rim is very strong and is usually spared any injury. The eye socket walls surrounded by sinuses are weak, particularly the floor. Compression from the trauma causes swelling and pushes the contents through the floor trapping them in the maxillary sinus. This results in: swelling, ecchymosis & diplopia with limited EOM movements, particularly the upward gaze.

1   orbital fossa
2   floor of the orbit
3   trapped contents - includes fat, IO, IR
4   maxillary sinus
5   bony fragments

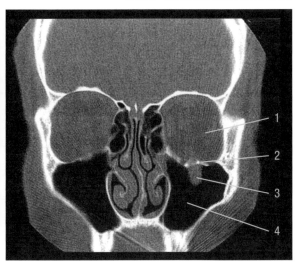

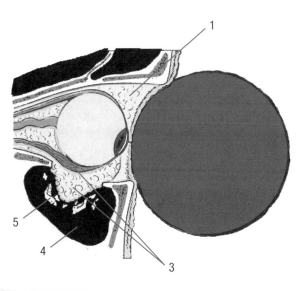

Visual Acuity (VA)

VA is the assessment of visual ability to discriminate object details & shapes. There are several ways in which this can be measured.

Distant VA is measured by a Snellen chart or equivalent (e.g. LogMAR chart, rolling E chart & shapes for children etc) using the smallest identifiable image that can be distinguished at 6m / 20ft. The numerator is the distance away from the chart - 6m. The denominator is the lowest height of the of letter (or shape) which can be distinguished at that distance 6cm.

VA Level	Description
6/6	Normal vision
6/12	Reduced vision, (Australian legal driving limit)
6/18	Low vision (World Health Organisation definition)
6/60	Legal blindness (eligible for entitlements)

When VA is too reduced to see a chart, the following terms are used:

Term	Description
CF	count fingers at distance specified
HM	Hand movement - at a close distance in front of the eyes
LP	Light Perception - only light & dark can be perceived - no details
NLP	No light perception - totally blind

Near VA tests a person's central vision. It is recorded in point notation, the same as for computer font, and marked with an 'N'.

- N18 - N16 is large print
- N18 is 18 point font
- N8 is newsprint
- N6 is telephone book print

These are uncorrected VA measurements - i.e. VA w/o visual aids.

Best corrected VA - tests the maximum VA achievable with visual aids e.g. corrective lenses etc ~90% of people > 60yo < 80yo can achieve 6/6 best corrected VA

Visual Acuity (VA)
Age changes - Presbyopia

The commonest change in VA with age is the development of Presbyopia, resulting from a diminished ability of the lens to change its curvature.

Pure presbyopia can be corrected with simple magnifying lenses, which may be determined by the following chart.

DIOPTER	WEAK		MEDIUM				STRONG		
	+1.25	+1.50	+1.75	+2.00	+2.25	+2.50	+2.75	+3.25	+3.50
	If you can read this clearly, you need to select this. If you can read	If you can read this clearly, you need to select this. If you can	If you can read this clearly, you need to select this. If you	If you can read this clearly, you need to select this. If	If you can read this clearly, you need to	If you can read this clearly, you	If you can read this clearly,	If you can read this	If you can read this

Visual Acuity (VA)

Astigmatism

Irregularities in the cornea &/or lens will result changes in the astigmatic VA

Charts are used to detect this based on:

grating - ability to distinguish the presence of grating - i.e. alternative light & dark stripes
(this is one of the first forms of VA to deteriorate with age) often referred to as the astigmatic clock - in the normal eye looks even but variations are seen with astigmatism

minimum perceptible - degree to which a person can detect small dots, lines or patterns

minimum separable - degree to which a person can distinguish the presence of 2 separate objects placed close together (when they can be seen as 2 not 1)

vernier - ability to detect minute line misalignments

Colour & Contrast perception

The level of any VA may change with colour, particularly if there is macular involvement where there is the highest concentration of Cone cells & 50% of the Visual input is derived from.

Rods are concentrated in the peripheral region of the retina. They detect movement & contrast. Charts with a series of parallel &/or concentric grey lines (Arden plates) are used to determine the **contrast VA**.

Measurement of colour blindness is undertaken via colour plates with hidden figures w/n the many dotted circles, and different to these measures.

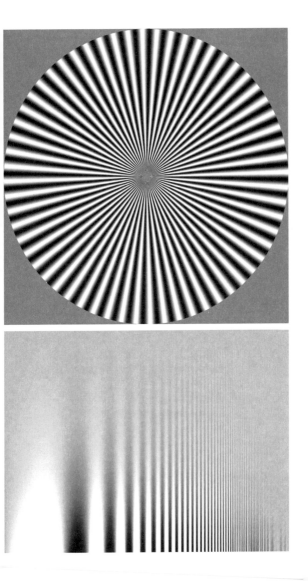

Visual Acuity Assessment
Amsler grid

There are several ways of assessing the VA - one of the most versatile is the Amsler grid.

This is a grid of evenly spaced vertical and horizontal lines with a central dark spot.

Although traditionally shown in black & white, there are other more sensitive colour version in particular the Blue / yellow Amsler. Results from the black & white Amsler may vary with a coloured chart particularly if rod cell pathology is involved..

Closing one eye and using whatever are the patient's usual visual aids the patient focuses on the central point for 30sec. This is then repeated with the other eye. In the normal eye the grid appears even.

If any changes are seen they are indicative of retinal &/or refractive changes in that eye.

1 Distortion - indicative of astigmatism, particularly thickened or thinned lines

2 White missing areas - indicative of scotomas - if small and multiple - indicative of DM retinopathy

3 Blurry semi-visible shape - fixed indicative of retinal detachment (RD)
   moving before settling in an area - indicative of floaters (often a prelude to RD)

4 Different shapes - indicative of rod cell displacement if in the periphery
   - indicative of cone cell displacement if more centrally placed, which may indicate a retinal fold

5 Central blackened area - indicative of MD

6 Double lines / diplopia - with the single eye this is indicative of early cataract formation

7 Rounding of the corners - i.e. not able to see the full square - indicative of peripheral VL most commonly seen in glaucoma

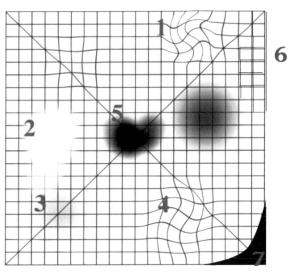

Visual Changes

EYE SYMPTOMS	COMMON DIAGNOSES
Acute spontaneous transient loss of vision in ONE EYE (Amaurosis Fugax)	1 Transient Ischaemia - CRAO or AV Hg 2 Migraine 3 Temporal Arteritis 4 ↑IOP
Acute spontaneous transient loss of vision in TWO EYES	1 TIA - affecting VP & / or Visual cortex 2 Migraine 3 ↑IOP
Lightning Flashes Streaks	1 Migraine 2 Retinal tears / detachment 3 Tugs on the retina by the VB
Blurred Vision - far sight / near sight	Myopia / Hyperopia
Diplopia / Double vision ONE EYE	1 Cataract 2 Lens detachment
Diplopia / Double vision TWO EYES	1 N &/or EOM damage 2 Entrapment of the EOM
Vertigo	Vestibular dysfunction
Loss of Central Vision ONE EYE	1 Glaucoma 2 Hysteria 3 drug toxicity
Loss of Side vision (lateral) TWO EYES	1 Lesion in the Optic Tract 2 lesion in the Optic Radiation
Loss of Night Vision TWO EYES	1 Retinosa Pigmentosa 2 Vitamin A deficiency 3 Cataract
Halos around lights	1 Cataract 2 Glaucoma

EYE SYMPTOMS	COMMON DIAGNOSES
Itching / Burning	1 Allergy 2 Conjunctivitis 3 Corneal irritation 4 FB 5 Dry Eyes
Pain with pressure on the EB	1 EL or orbital If 2 Scleritis / Episcleritis 3 Anterior Uveitis 4 Acute Angle Glaucoma
Photophobia	1 RE 2 If of eye adnexae 3 Migraine / Tension Headache 4 Sinusitis 5 Glaucoma 6 Uveitis 7 Cerebral Lesion 8 Hypertension

Visual Fields
Defects

Schema

Pressures at different point along the VP will result in diagnostic VF defects.

L column represents the view from the L eye

R column represents the view from the R eye

1. pressure on the L Optic N causes circumferential blindness on L side - the ipsilateral side
2. total blindness on the affected side of the cut CN II
3. pressure on the L optic tract results in R sided nasal hemianopia
4. pressure / lesions on the chiasm (as in pituitary tumors) result in bilateral temporal hemianopia – no side vision
5. L temporal hemianopia + R nasal hemianopia is the
6. result from lesions in the optic tract (5), Optic radiation
7. (6,9) and or in the Visual cortex (7,8)
8. visual cortex
9. optic radiation
10. lateral geniculate body
11. chiasm
12. CN II = ON
13. nasal bridge

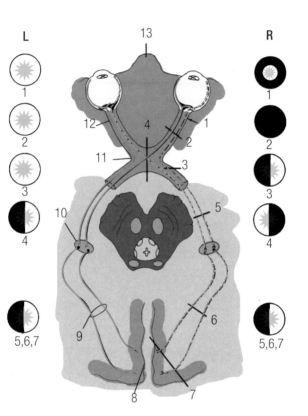

L

1

2

3

4

5,6,7

R

1

2

3

4

5,6,7

13

12

4

11

10

9

8

1

2

3

5

6

7

Visual Pathway

Sagittal view - cut through the middle of the brain
Transverse view - slice along the brain base
Schema of the process of bifocal vision & visual projections

The axons of the retina coalesce at the back of the eye at the OD - blind spot and move through the optic canal at the posterior of the orbit, as the ON (2). At the chiasm (3) 50% of the N fibres cross to the contralateral side & leave as the optic tract (4) and synapse in the lateral geniculate body (5). They emerge as the optic radiation (6), which travels to the visual cortex (7) - Brodman's areas 17, 18 & 19 in the Occipital lobe (14) either side of the Calcarine sulcus (15).

Because of the different positions of the eyes, each eye has a slightly different view of an image. These 2 images are able to be reconciled in the brain and give an impression of depth, distance & relative position.

1   retina
      p = projection on the retina
2   ON
3   chiasm
4   optic tract
5   lateral geniculate body
      p = projection on the nucleus
6   optic radiation
7   visual cortex
8   corona radiata
9   brainstem
10 superior colliculus
11 pulvinar (of the thalamus)
12 medial geniculate body
13 mammillary body
14 occipital lobe - with striate cortex
      p = projection on the striate cortex
15 calcarine sulcus

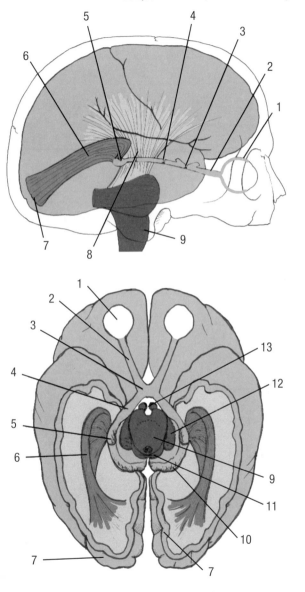

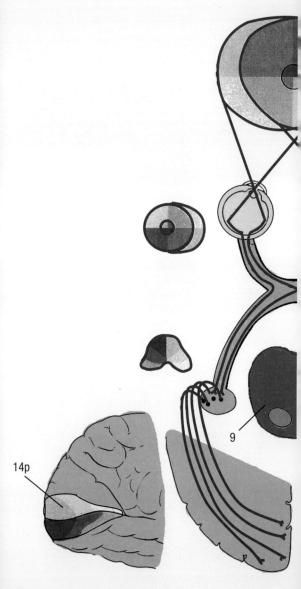

14p

9

© A. L. Neill

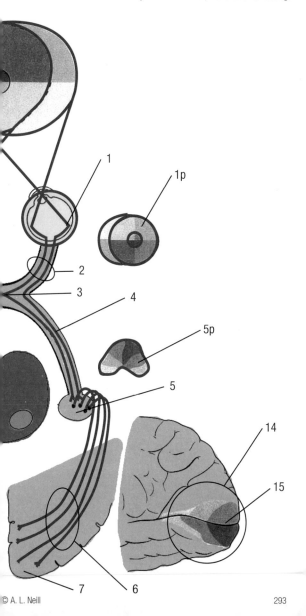

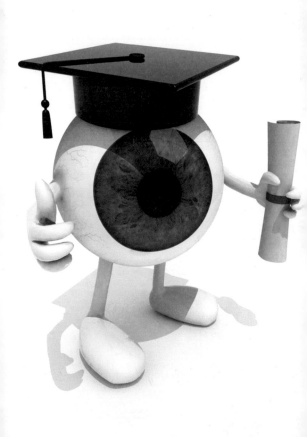